Why Can't Anyone Help Me?

The Nightmare of Adenomyosis

ISBN-13: 978-1986645676
ISBN-10: 1986645673

Cover design by Heidi Sutherlin, www.mycreativepursuits.com

Important notices:

Many of the supplements in this book have not been evaluated by the U.S. Food and Drug Administration. The supplements and statements in this book are not intended to diagnose, treat, cure or prevent adenomyosis, endometriosis or any other disease. The author accepts no responsibility for any illness or harm as a result of the use or misuse of the supplements described in this book.

The recommendations in this book are based on the author's own research of clinical studies. The author is not a physician. This book is not intended as a substitute for the medical advice of a physician. The reader should regularly consult with a physician in matters relating to her health and particularly with respect to any symptoms that may require diagnosis or medical attention.

Although the author and publisher have made every effort to ensure that the information in this book was correct at press time, the author and publisher do not assume and hereby disclaim any liability to any party for any loss, damage or disruption caused by errors or omissions, whether such errors or omissions result from negligence, accident or any other cause.

Table of Contents

Preface

I can't even tell you the number of times I have heard "Why can't anyone help me?" when it comes to dealing with the uterine disorder adenomyosis. As the founder of the online group Adenomyosis Fighters, my heart breaks each time I hear those words. Having suffered from the pain and discomfort of this disorder for seventeen years and after years of trying to promote more education and research on this disorder, I still can't effectively answer that question. Although some progress has been made, we still have a very long way to go to understand the specifics on the development and treatment of adenomyosis.

Some physicians are as frustrated as I am regarding this subject. I know of one physician who, when given my book, just shook his head and said, "That disorder is almost impossible to diagnose and treat." However, this physician was happy to receive the book. I wish more physicians would be as receptive.

Other physicians and even media personalities tout misinformation. Several years ago, a physician suggested on his radio show that there was no evidence that endometriosis, a similar disorder, was a physical problem. Instead, he suggested that it stemmed from a psychological issue and a history of abuse. This information is not only insulting for those of us that deal with adenomyosis, but it also sets us back in terms of finding the real cause and effective treatments for this uterine disorder.

Recent studies have shown that magnetic resonance imaging, or MRI, might be an effective way to diagnose this condition. However, to this day, I still hear stories of how physicians are telling their patients that the only way to diagnose adenomyosis is through hysterectomy. These antiquated beliefs are a result of physicians not keeping up with the current knowledge. I was even stunned the other day when I read a post on my support group site. Her physician told her that adenomyosis doesn't cause any pain! That statement is false, and it goes to show that adenomyosis patients must "shop around" to find top physicians that are up-to-date on the current knowledge of this disorder.

My previous book, *Adenomyosis: A Significantly Neglected and Misunderstood Uterine Disorder*, was a general overview of the disorder and a review of the scientific studies completed at that time. This new book is a much more in-depth look at this disorder, including detailed information the functioning of the female reproductive tract, the role of hormones, current diagnostic procedures and treatments, the role of estrogen dominance and xenoestrogens, diet and supplement tips, and how stress can induce hormonal imbalance leading to the development of the disorder. The role of phytoestrogens, a controversial topic, is discussed in detail. In this book, I have even included a section on the emotional aspects of this disorder as anxiety and depression play a major role in this disorder.

Note: Although adenomyosis is the focus of this book, I will also discuss endometriosis at times. There is a good reason for this. In many cases, endometriosis occurs along with adenomyosis, so it is important to have information on both disorders especially if you are about to undergo a hysterectomy. As you will read later in this book, hysterectomy is a cure for adenomyosis, but it is not a cure for endometriosis. Therefore, if you have a hysterectomy for adenomyosis but have continuing pain after surgery, you might also have endometriosis.

I hope that this book helps to pave the way to better education, diagnosis and treatments for those suffering from this nightmare of a uterine disorder.

Introduction

For A Moment, Imagine the Pain

For the next few minutes, I ask you to put yourself in another person's shoes. Just imagine.

Imagine waking up in the middle of the night to excruciating pain that comes in waves, first in your lower abdomen and then moving to your lower back. These waves of pain come every three to four minutes and are similar to full stage labor pains or kidney stone pain.

Imagine not knowing the reason or cause of this pain.

Imagine that you have no way to control this pain. The doctors have given you all kinds of medication, but nothing works.

Imagine going through this pain for five to six hours during an attack...waves of intense pain every three to four minutes which then start to move down to the upper parts of your legs. You could swear you are giving birth.

Imagine standing at the bathroom sink with sweat pouring off your face and horrible nausea due to the terrible waves of pain. You can't stand up straight because the pain is so unbearable.

Imagine holding onto the sides of the bathroom sink as you try not to faint as yet another wave of pain hits you. You see stars, and you try to position yourself so that you won't hit your head if you fall.

Imagine an intense wave of pain throughout your belly as you grab onto the toilet to vomit...multiple times.

Imagine lying on the bathroom floor in the fetal position as you cry out of frustration while you are forced to endure this nightmare.

Imagine having menstrual periods that last ten to fourteen days per month with spotting on other days.

Imagine having so much blood loss that you soak a maxi pad in an hour.

Imagine how tired you feel because of the chronic anemia.

Imagine that you pass blood clots that are as big as the palm of your hand.

Imagine that you have so much abdominal bloating that you look three to four months pregnant.

Now imagine that this happens to you at least once a month.

Imagine trying to get pregnant while enduring all of this, but it never happens. You never have children.

Imagine the anxiety that you feel because you never know when an attack will hit you. You make sure you are always close to a bathroom. You panic as you drive down the highway and start to feel pelvic pain.

Imagine going through this while trying to hold down a full-time job. What will your boss or co-workers say when you take another sick day?

Imagine trying to be a parent while suffering from this uterine disorder. You can't take a sick day as a parent.

Imagine that you undergo numerous invasive tests only to be told that they can't find the cause of your problems.

Imagine being told that you need to see a psychologist because of this problem, and you are put on antidepressant medication for your depression and anxiety.

Imagine your friends, acquaintances and "experts" telling you that it's "all in your head" because the doctors can't find the cause of your pain.

Imagine going through multiple surgeries but the pain and heavy bleeding always return.

Imagine having an endometrial ablation and being told that this surgery will certainly stop the bleeding. The bleeding returns twenty-four hours after surgery.

Imagine having a hysterectomy before finally obtaining a correct diagnosis...after years of unbearable physical, mental and emotional pain. It was adenomyosis.

Imagine a doctor telling you that he doesn't know anything about adenomyosis. He tells you to "google" it.

Just imagine...
Imagine the frustration.
Imagine the pain.
Imagine your quality of life during that time.

Imagine...

My Adenomyosis Story

The following is a copy of a blog that is published on the Adenomyosis Fighter's website. It gives a summary of my seventeen-year ordeal with this disorder. Although I no longer have any symptoms thanks to my hysterectomy, I am so passionate about helping other women who are forced to deal with this horrible uterine disorder because I can deeply empathize with their pain.

As I continue to push for more education and research for adenomyosis, I am so affected by all the stories that I read from women who are currently struggling with this uterine disorder. I read a lot of posts by women who just want basic information. These women are desperate to know that there are other women out there who are going through the same thing. Therefore, I have decided to write a blog post on my experience, hoping that this information will help others who are currently suffering with adenomyosis.

From the first day of my first menstrual period at the age of 14, I have had bad cramps and heavy bleeding. I remember coming home from high school because I was in so much pain and taking Motrin to stop the cramps. I was told that this was all normal. All women have cramps and feel like hell during their periods. It was all just a part of being a woman.

When I went to college, I noticed that a lot of the girls in my dorm just seemed to breeze through that time of the month. Although it wasn't a main topic of discussion, it seemed like some girls never had low energy...ever. They always felt pretty good and had so much more energy than I did. I really began to blame myself for not being a stronger woman. Why did I struggle so much during "that time of the month"? I was drained, moody, and had

19

horrible headaches that didn't seem to respond to ibuprofen. I began to refer to these headaches as "menstrual headaches".

The real nightmare started in 1990. I woke up one morning to searing abdominal pain. Now, for comparison, I had a ruptured appendix in 1986, and obviously, I clearly remember that pain. The surgeon told me that I was very close to death after my appendectomy as my appendix was also gangrenous. I ended up with peritonitis (a very serious abdominal infection) and was on IV antibiotics for six days. My surgeon told me that if I ever felt pain like that again, I needed to get to the hospital as soon as possible. I never forgot that.

Back to the morning in 1990 – this abdominal pain was even more severe than the pain I felt from the ruptured appendix! It came in waves every few minutes, and when the pain hit, I thought I was going to pass out. Sweat poured down my face, and by the time the attack was over, my shirt was soaking wet. I felt like I had to have a bowel movement, but I was unable to defecate. At the time, I had just finished my period, which was horribly heavy and long (about ten days), and I was still spotting. I was petrified! I called my mom, and she came to pick me up to go to the hospital. I told her that I was in so much pain that I couldn't even walk to the car, but she helped me, and somehow, I made it. As I compared this to the experience with the ruptured appendix, I was sure that I was on my death bed.

When I arrived at the hospital, I felt like I needed to have a bowel movement again. I raced to the bathroom and had a huge bout of diarrhea. I felt a little bit better, but those waves of pain kept coming. The ER doctor ran a bunch of tests, but they all came back normal. He gave me some narcotic pain meds through an IV and told me I probably had food poisoning. He sent me home. I must *admit that I was a bit skeptical. This pain was more severe than the pain I felt after my ruptured appendix. Was this really food poisoning, or did he miss something?*

Other than painful menstrual cramps, lengthy periods, and spotting, nothing really happened for about a year. During that time, I married and continued to work while continuing to put up with these difficult menstrual cycles. Then, suddenly, I awoke one night to the exact same abdominal pain. I sweated profusely, had excruciating cramping pain that doubled me over every few minutes, felt like I was going to pass out from the pain, and became very nauseated. Again, I felt like I needed to defecate but was unable to do so. After about five hours and having yet another bout of profuse diarrhea, things settled down. This attack also happened at the very end of my menstrual period, and I was spotting at the time. I called in sick to work the next day, and I went to the doctor.

After explaining that this exact same thing had happened twice, the doctor was concerned that I had irritable bowel syndrome. He ordered a colonoscopy. Well, the colonoscopy came back completely normal. In fact, the gastroenterologist said that my colon looked so good that I didn't need to have another colonoscopy for twenty years! I was frustrated. What was causing this horrendous pain?

As the years went by, these attacks became more frequent. They mostly occurred at the end of my menstrual period which clued me into the fact that this could be a gynecological problem. However, when I went to my gynecologist, he assured me that everything was normal and just told me to take ibuprofen. I was told that this was all "normal".

My co-workers began to doubt that I was sick. People began to talk behind my back. Since the doctors couldn't find anything wrong with me, they assumed that I was a hypochondriac.

My worst year was 1996. I had these attacks AT LEAST once a month, and all of them occurred before, during, or at the end of my menstrual period. I decided to change gynecologists and get a second opinion. I traveled to a teaching hospital in Georgia at the recommendation of a friend, and I was super optimistic that I would get an answer there. This gynecologist scheduled a laparoscopy to investigate the cause of the pain. The surgery identified some endometriosis which was ablated during the procedure, and I hoped that this would finally be the answer. However, it wasn't. Two months after surgery, the pain returned full force.

I returned to this doctor several more times, but she was unable to find the underlying cause of the issue. The attacks continued and even worsened. I remember several nights in particular. One night, the pain was so severe that I was having diarrhea while vomiting in the trash can at the same time. On another night, the most severe cramp that I had ever had came across my abdomen, and I literally thought my intestine was going to rupture. On yet another night, I saw stars when a cramp hit me, and I thought for sure I was going to faint. I just grabbed onto the sink and told myself to breathe as I positioned myself so I wouldn't hit my head if I fell. I remember lying on the bathroom floor in the fetal position, crying out of extreme frustration, begging God to deliver me from this nightmare. With each attack, I always felt like I had to have a bowel movement, but I couldn't go. Some nights, I would become so frustrated that I would push as hard as I could, desperately trying to defecate. This led to the development of hemorrhoids.

Over the years, I noticed that I would become extremely bloated just prior to the attack. In fact, if people didn't *know any better, they would think I was pregnant. Once the bloating began, I knew I was in trouble and that I better get home as soon as possible. I also began to pass incredibly large blood clots, some as big as the palm of my hand. I KNEW that this had to be some kind of gynecological disorder.*

I began to have panic attacks. If I started to bloat or started to feel any kind of pelvic pain and I wasn't at home, my heart would race, and I would start to feel faint. I would begin to shake and feel panicky, especially if I wasn't near a bathroom. I remember a trip that my husband and I took to Las Vegas, and when we were in the airport to catch our flight home, I began to bloat. I became shaky and nauseated, and I began to have pelvic pain as we waited in line for our tickets. I went to the bathroom since I felt like I needed to defecate, but I couldn't. Panic overtook me, and we had to stay in Vegas an additional two days before I could travel home. The doctor who I saw in Vegas was convinced that I had gastroesophageal reflux which I knew was a bunch of nonsense. Honestly, I wanted to tell him off because he wasn't listening to me, but I was just too sick. He did give me some medication that made me sleep, and this is really what it took to get me home. I don't think I would have traveled had I not been sedated.

Eventually, we moved to Virginia. I searched for a well-respected gynecologist and again had some hope when I found one that was highly recommended. I told her all that had happened to me, and she ran all the tests that had already been run on me in Georgia. Of course, everything came back normal. She suggested that I try birth control pills. These helped a little bit, but I still was miserable and still had the occasional attacks of severe pain.

23

I went back to her repeatedly, and I could tell that she was becoming increasingly impatient with me during each visit. One time, I went with a detailed list of my symptoms and when I experienced them. As I started to read the list to explain things to her, she grabbed it from me, glanced at it a few seconds, and then threw it on the chair. As she performed my exam, I tried to ask her more questions, but I could tell she wasn't interested in helping me. She told me, "I have to go. I have other naked women waiting on me".

Extremely frustrated, I went to yet another gynecologist that was recommended to me. This guy was worse than the other gynecologist. He actually closed his eyes while I talked to him, and I could swear he was dozing. He did all the routine tests, the same as the other doctors, and couldn't find any problems.

I continued to try to live my life as normally as possible. I had been prescribed a slew of different medications over the years, and none of them worked. At one point, I was prescribed Bentyl for irritable bowel syndrome, and this medication was completely useless. When one of the attacks started, I took that medication immediately with high hopes of it at least lessening the pain. This medication did absolutely nothing...no pain relief at all, and that attack ended up being one of the most severe attacks I ever had. Most of the doctors wanted to jump to the conclusion that I had IBS since they couldn't find anything else. It is important to note that IBS is a diagnosis of exclusion. This means that if all other tests are negative, they assign the label of "IBS". To me, this basically means that they don't know the real cause of the problem.

Finally, out of desperation, I looked to natural alternatives. I read up on the benefits of flaxseed, and I was intrigued. I began to incorporate ground flaxseed (very high in omega-3 fatty acids) into my diet, and my symptoms improved dramatically. I was amazed! This propelled me into alternative medicine which led to my Master's degree in Holistic Nutrition.

Although dietary changes did bring some relief, I still struggled with prolonged menstrual bleeding that lasted up to fourteen day at this point in my life, spotting for several days after that, bad menstrual cramps, digestive problems during menstruation, passing extremely large blood clots, infertility (we tried for ten years with no confirmed pregnancy), menstrual migraine headaches, and terrible PMS (mood swings in particular). I was eventually diagnosed with a uterine polyp via hysterosonogram. The actual procedure was not bad at all (I expected it to be painful). However, on our way home (about 15-20 minutes later), severe cramping started. We were stuck in horrible traffic, and I told my husband to pull over. The car next to us wouldn't let us over which obviously made both of us mad. I thought I was going to vomit from the pain, but there was nothing my husband could do. Finally, we were able to pull into a McDonald's restaurant. Making it to the bathroom just in time, I had a huge bout of diarrhea which lessened the pain enough that I could get home. After this experience, I was convinced that my uterus was the problem. The polyp was removed through hysteroscopy, but even after this surgery, the symptoms continued.

Several years later, we moved to Texas. Finally, I came across a gynecologist who was empathetic to my situation. She suggested that I have an endometrial ablation to see if that would ease my symptoms, and I agreed to do so. This surgery is supposed to stop all bleeding as it burns the endometrial lining of the uterus. However, 24 hours after surgery, I began to bleed. Since this isn't supposed to happen, I went to the hospital.

Emergency room physicians are sometimes not very good at performing gynecological exams as I found out during this trip to the ER. During the exam, I was torn which caused me even more pain. I was fuming mad, and I can't even describe the amount of stress and frustration that I felt at the time. Of course, the ER doctors couldn't find any problem other than I was bleeding when I shouldn't be bleeding. A lot of good that trip did for me!

The next day, I went back to see my gynecologist. When she examined me, she was very concerned. I remember her words: "Wow, this is way too much bleeding. This has never happened with any other ablation that I have done." At that time, I asked for a hysterectomy, and she agreed.

I really was quite happy on the day of the hysterectomy in 2007. Finally, this uterus that has put me through hell is going to come out! The ovaries were left as I was still in my early forties, and my gynecologist didn't want me to go into early menopause.

The follow-up visit with my gynecologist is one day I will never forget. She came into the room and FINALLY explained to me why I had so much pain over all those years. I had severe diffuse adenomyosis with fibroids. She went on to explain that this condition cannot be definitively diagnosed prior to hysterectomy and that it could explain all my issues over the past seventeen years. Needless to say, I couldn't have been happier. The next day, I sent her flowers, thanking her for finally identifying the cause of my pain.

Since my hysterectomy, ALL of my symptoms have completely resolved. I have not had any attacks since that day.

What is Adenomyosis?

Adenomyosis is a uterine disorder that can cause a whole host of problems including painful and prolonged menstruation, heavy bleeding, and an enlarged uterus. A comprehensive list of all the symptoms can be found in Chapter 7. It can dramatically reduce the quality of a woman's life because of the excruciating pain, fatigue, anemia from excessive blood loss, and emotional pain associated with fertility issues. It is known to be an estrogen-dependent disorder (Yamanaka et al., 2014).

In Chapter 1, we will get into a more detailed discussion of the female reproductive tract. For now, to explain it in simple terms, the uterus has two main layers – the endometrium and the myometrium. The endometrium is the inner layer and responds to hormonal stimulation. The buildup of the endometrium is shed each month in the form of a menstrual period. The myometrium is the outer uterine muscle that contracts during childbirth and menstruation. In a normal uterus, these layers are distinct and separate. However, in adenomyosis, for unknown reasons, the endometrium invades the myometrium. During menstruation, these endometrial implants within the myometrium respond to hormonal stimulation and they literally bleed into the uterine muscle which can cause extreme pain. This condition was first described by Rokitansky in 1860 and von Recklinghausen in 1896 (Benagiano, Brosens, Carrara, & Filippi, 2010).

Adenomyosis can be "focal" (localized to one area) or "diffuse" (spread throughout the entire uterine muscle). The "focal" form of adenomyosis is referred to as an adenomyoma, and it is fairly easy to detect because it can usually be identified on imaging studies. However, an adenomyoma many times can be confused with a fibroid. "Diffuse" adenomyosis is much more difficult to detect; hence the problem with diagnosis. In addition, adenomyosis can involve the entire thickness of the myometrium. Usually the posterior wall of the uterus is the most severely affected. It differs from fibroids in that adenomyosis does not have clear, distinct borders. This makes removal of the adenomyotic tissue very difficult if not impossible.

Adenomyosis throughout the uterine wall causes irregular and inefficient uterine contractions. As a result, the uterine contractions are not able to contract around the large blood vessels that feed the endometrium. This is the main cause for prolonged and heavy bleeding in this disorder.

The following are some interesting statistic about this disorder:

1. 80% of women with this disorder also have other uterine lesions with fibroids being the most common. As previously stated, it is very difficult to differentiate between fibroids and adenomyomas.
2. 50% of women with adenomyosis also have fibroids (Garavaglia et al., 2015).
3. Polyps and adenocarcinoma occur more frequently in women with adenomyosis. In addition, a study by Choi et al. (2017) has shown that benign ovarian tumors, anemia and high cholesterol levels are seen more frequently in women with adenomyosis and endometriosis.
4. According to Garavaglia et al. (2015), 70% of women with adenomyosis also have endometriosis. This is important to know since many women who undergo a hysterectomy for adenomyosis continue to have pain. Since a hysterectomy cures adenomyosis through the removal of the uterus, continuing pain after hysterectomy is usually an indication of the presence of endometriosis.
5. According to Garavaglia et al. (2015), 35% of women with adenomyosis also have endometrial hyperplasia.
6. 60% of women with endometrial carcinoma also have adenomyosis.

Adenomyosis has previously been reported to primarily affect middle-aged women and women who have had children. However, this line of thinking is beginning to change as more women are reporting symptoms of adenomyosis at a younger age and in those without children. In fact, according to Garavaglia et al. (2015), the pathological events in adenomyosis can appear in adolescence.

Current diagnosis of this disorder prior to surgery is low, ranging from 3% to 26% (Taran, Stewart & Brucker, 2013). The cause of this disorder is currently unknown as is the prevalence. Due to the lack of knowledge on this disorder, prevalence has been reported to be from 5% to 70% (Taran et al., 2013). At hysterectomy, the reported cases are around 20 to 30% (Taran et al., 2013). Additionally, according to Bromley, Shipp and Benacerraf (2000), "the symptoms are so non-specific that the diagnosis is made preoperatively in fewer than half of patients undergoing hysterectomy" (Discussion section, para. 2).

Adenomyosis is asymptomatic in about one-third of cases. The disorder may be found incidentally by ultrasound or during a hysterectomy. According to Garavaglia et al. (2015), "in these cases, diagnosis can be also mistaken from 10-90% among pathologists if histological criteria are not strictly followed."

Now that you have a very basic understanding of adenomyosis, let's delve more deeply into the specifics of this disorder.

This book is divided into five sections. Section 1 will explain the basics of the female reproductive tract. Although some readers may find this part uninteresting, it is important to have a basic understanding of how the reproductive tract works along with the functions of hormones in the female body in order to understand how and why adenomyosis and endometriosis develops.

Section II will get into more specifics on adenomyosis and endometriosis. I include endometriosis because these two disorders often occur together. Fibroids and uterine polyps will also be addressed in this section as these disorders are also seen more often in women with adenomyosis. Ongoing scientific studies into potential causes of this disorder will be examined as well as diagnostic tests and current treatments.

Section III will discuss estrogen dominance and how this plays into the development of adenomyosis. Xenoestrogens (chemicals in the environment that act like estrogen) are discussed at length.

Section IV covers diet, herbs and other supplements that may help control the disorder. A review of phytoestrogens and the role of omega-3 fatty acids in symptom reduction is addressed in this section.

Section V covers the emotional aspects of dealing with adenomyosis and how stress can exacerbate symptoms.

Current ongoing studies, recommended reading, recommended physicians, abbreviations, and definitions finish out the book. If, while you are reading this book, you forget what an acronym stands for, you can refer to the abbreviation section to get a quick refresher. There are quite a few acronyms used in scientific studies and throughout this book, and sometimes it is hard to keep them straight!

I hope you find this book helpful as you deal with this incredibly difficult uterine disorder.

Section I

Chapter 1 - Basics of the Female Reproductive Tract

"Yet over two decades of my practice, it has become clear to me that healing cannot occur for women until we have critically examined and changed some of the beliefs and assumptions that we all unconsciously inherit and internalize from our culture."

-Christiane Northrup, MD, from her book, Women's Bodies, Women's Wisdom

Before I get into a more in-depth discussion of adenomyosis, it is important that we understand the basics of the female reproductive tract. In the next few chapters, I will review the anatomy of the reproductive tract along with an in-depth discussion of hormones and how each one works. I will also discuss how hormonal balance is extremely important to the proper functioning of the reproductive tract. If you take the time to learn these basics, you will more clearly understand how adenomyosis develops and how hormonal imbalance causes much of the discomfort of the disorder.

The uterus is located between the urinary bladder and the rectum. It is divided into three different parts: the fundus, the body of the uterus and the cervix. The uterus is about 8 cm. long, 5 cm. wide and 4 cm. thick (Behera & Gest, 2011), and it is supported within the pelvis by broad ligaments. Within the body of the uterus, there are three distinct layers:

- The inner layer consists of glandular mucosa and is called the endometrium. This layer responds to the action of follicle-stimulating hormone (FSH) and luteinizing hormone (LH) surges from the anterior pituitary gland. This layer also consists of two individual layers – the stratus functionalis and the stratus basalis. The stratum functionalis is involved in the thickening of this layer each month and is shed in the form of a menstrual period. This layer grows under the influence of estrogen and progesterone from the corpus luteum, a structure formed after the release of an egg each month. The stratum basalis is unresponsive to the cyclical hormonal levels.

- The thick and muscular middle layer is called the myometrium and contains bundles of smooth muscle that contract rhythmically. This is the largest layer of the uterus and is the powerful muscular layer that contract during childbirth and menstruation. It is regulated by oxytocin, prostaglandins and the autonomic nervous system.

- The outer layer is called the perimetrium (also referred to as the serosa layer). This layer envelops the uterus and consists of epithelial cells.

In addition to the above three layers, a distinct area can be seen between the endometrium and myometrium on magnetic resonance imaging (MRI). This area is called the junctional zone or JZ.

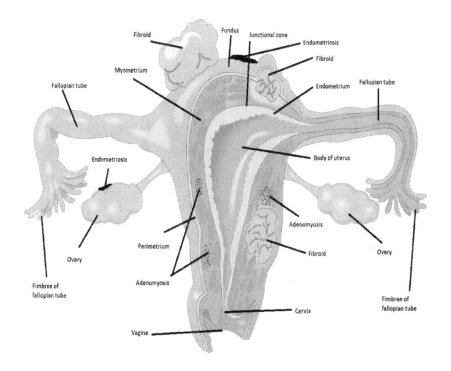

Blood is supplied to the uterus through the uterine artery. This artery branches off into smaller arteries called radial arteries. The radial arteries supply blood to the myometrium and the endometrium. In the endometrium, they branch off even further to form basal and spiral arteries. The spiral arteries respond to female hormone levels, and when conception does not occur, these little arteries constrict resulting in a menstrual period.

The uterus can also have varying positions within the pelvis. Sometimes the uterus tilts forward (anteflexion) or tilts backward (retroflexion). The anteflexed position is considered normal. The retroflexed position is considered a normal variant and supposedly doesn't cause any reproductive issues. Additionally, the uterus may also vary in size. During puberty and the post-menopausal years, the uterus may be smaller than during childbearing years. It may also be smaller in women who have had no children in comparison to those who have given birth.

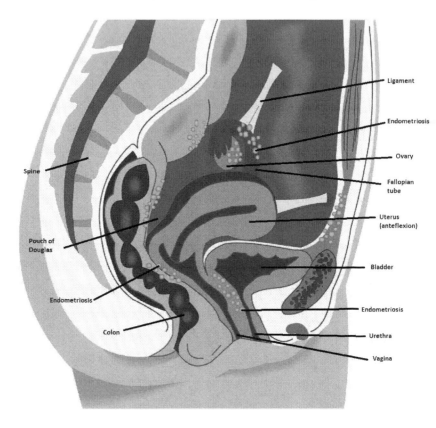

In addition to adenomyosis and endometriosis, there are other abnormalities that can occur in the uterus. The following is a list of some of these abnormalities along with a quick description of the problem. Some of these disorders have been seen in conjunction with adenomyosis.

Arcuate uterus – In this condition, the uterus has a slight indentation at the top. This is considered a normal uterine variant with no known adverse effects.

Asheman syndrome – In this syndrome, scarring inside the uterus occurs due to infection or surgery. Adhesions may be present.

Bicornuate uterus – This disorder is seen in about 1 out of every 200 women. Also called a "heart-shaped" uterus, this results from the failure of the upper part of the Mullerian ducts to fuse during development which leaves the upper portion of the uterus divided into two sections. A bicornuate uterus does not appear to have any adverse effects on pregnancy.

Endometrial hyperplasia – Seen in women with adenomyosis, this is a condition where there is overgrowth of the endometrium.

Endometrial cancer – This form of cancer arises from the endometrial lining of the uterus.

Incompetent cervix – In this disorder, the cervix dilates too soon during pregnancy which results in pre-term labor or second trimester pregnancy loss.

Septate uterus – This is the most common congenital (present from birth) abnormality of the uterus. In this disorder, the uterus is divided partially or completely by a band of tissue or muscle. A septate uterus can result in repeat cases of miscarriage, but thankfully, it can be corrected through surgery. It is seen in about 1 out of 45 women.

Unicornuate uterus – In this disorder, only one half of the uterus forms. Only one fallopian tube and ovary are present. This rare disorder occurs in about 1 in every 1000 women.

Uterine cancer – Risk factors for this type of cancer include age over 50, obesity, taking unopposed estrogen (estrogen without progesterone) and family history of uterine cancer. Symptoms include an abnormal vaginal discharge, abnormal vaginal bleeding, pelvic pain and/or pelvic pressure.

Uterine didelphys – This disorder occurs when the Mullerian ducts fail to fuse during development and results in two separate uteri. Many times, there is also a separate cervix and vagina associated with each uterus. Also referred to as a double uterus, this disorder occurs in about 1 out of every 350 women.

Uterine fibroid – These are benign masses that form from the myometrium layer of the uterus and may be present in women with adenomyosis. A study by Shrestha and Sedai (2012) looked at the differences between women with adenomyosis alone and those with adenomyosis and uterine fibroids. They found women with adenomyosis only had higher levels of chronic pelvic pain and a smaller uterus. The women who had fibroids only had less pelvic pain and a larger uterus. They suggested that if a woman presents with fibroids, a small uterus and chronic pelvic pain, the physician should suspect the co-existence of adenomyosis with fibroids.

Uterine polyp – These benign growths are found inside the uterus and are due to the overgrowth of the endometrium. They may be present in women with adenomyosis.

The Ovaries

There are two ovaries, one on each side of the uterus. They are located in an area called the ovarian fossa. Each ovary is about 3.5 centimeters long, 1 centimeter thick and 2 centimeters wide. The ovaries are held in place by several ligaments: the broad ligament, the suspensory ligament and the ovarian ligament. Each ovary has an inner medulla and an outer cortex. The ovarian follicles that hold eggs are located in the outer cortex. The medulla contains mostly blood vessels, nerve fibers and connective tissue.

During fetal development, several million primordial follicles form, and each one contains a primary oocyte. Over the course of the life of a woman, a lot of these follicles with the oocytes degenerate. Only about 400 to 500 go on to be released from the ovary during a woman's lifetime.

The Fallopian Tubes

Two fallopian tubes, one on each side of the uterus, open into the uterus at its widest spot. The tubes are held in place by the broad ligament and are about 10 centimeters long and 0.7 centimeters in diameter. The top of the tube opens into a funnel-shaped region called the infundibulum which contain finger-like projections called fimbrae. The action of the cilia, peristaltic action and the mucous secreted by the epithelium in the tube helps the egg to travel down to the uterus.

The Cervix

The cervix is the lower one third of the uterus, and it connects the uterus to the vagina. The cervical canal can be broken down into the internal and external os. The internal os refers to the narrow portion of the canal that leads into the uterus. The myometrium in this region is thinner than the myometrium in the rest of the uterus. The external os refers to the opening where the cervix opens into the vagina. The external os is surrounded by cervical tissue, and it protrudes slightly into the vagina.

The cervix controls how and when substances move into and out of the uterus. Basically, this is done through mucous production. To prevent movement into and out of the uterus, thick mucus is formed into a mucous plug. During ovulation, the mucous thins out which makes it easier for sperm to enter the uterus.

The Vagina

About 9 centimeters long, the vagina is a muscular tube that connects the uterus to the outer part of the body. It typically extends upward and back in the pelvis and is located behind the bladder and in front of the rectum. Connective tissue connects bladder and rectum to the vagina; however, the upper fourth of the vagina is separated from the rectum. This region is known as the rectovaginal pouch, also known as the pouch of Douglas.

Chapter 2 - The Sex Hormones

"You can think of your body's many hormones as part of an elaborate messenger system, dashing through your bloodstream to share information, give instructions, and coordinate functions among your organs and nervous system."

-Marcelle Pick from her book, Is it Me or My Hormones?

The entire menstruation process begins in an organ at the base of the brain called the hypothalamus. Day one of a woman's cycle is the first day of bleeding. Low levels of estrogen and progesterone signal the hypothalamus to produce gonadotropin-releasing hormone, or GnRH. This hormone is sent to the pituitary gland (immediately underneath the hypothalamus) where, through stimulation by GnRH, follicle-stimulating hormone (FSH) is made and sent to the ovary. This is called the follicular phase of the menstrual cycle and lasts through the first half of the cycle. Increases in FSH cause anywhere from a few to several hundred follicles in the ovary to start producing estrogen. The oocyte in the follicle starts to mature, and when the oocyte separates from its surrounding granulosa cells, it becomes known as a primary follicle. When the oocyte is pushed to the side of the follicle because of the proliferation of follicular cells, it is then known as a secondary follicle. As many as twenty follicles mature during a cycle, but usually only one follicle outgrows all the other follicles. This one follicle is known as the dominant follicle, and as it develops, the other ones typically degenerate.

Meanwhile, the increase in estrogen causes the endometrial lining to grow and thicken in preparation for pregnancy. This thickened endometrium is engorged with blood which will serve to feed a growing fetus. Estrogen also softens the cervix, produces vaginal secretions and improves mood. At around day 10, the pituitary gland is stimulated by the high estrogen levels to produce luteinizing hormone (LH). This is the beginning of the ovulatory phase. At around day 12, the estrogen level peaks and then slowly begins to drop. At around day 14-15, a surge of LH causes the dominant follicle to rupture which releases an egg.

The egg is suspended in follicular fluid, and this fluid oozes toward the fallopian tube. This is known as ovulation, and at this time, the vaginal mucous becomes thin and clear and resembles uncooked egg whites. This change in mucous makes the environment more hospitable to sperm. The change in mucous consistency combined with a small rise in temperature caused by the increase in progesterone production is the optimum time for sexual activity if a pregnancy is desired. Once the egg is released, the cycle enters the luteal phase which lasts 12 to 14 days. The cilia inside the fallopian tube beat toward the uterus which helps the egg travel down the tube where it awaits fertilization. In the meantime, the remnants of the ovarian follicle develop into a small yellow body called the corpus luteum. This small structure produces progesterone which stops the buildup of the endometrium by counteracting the effects of estrogen. Progesterone is the dominant hormone during this time, and levels usually peak at about 20 mg per day. If the egg is fertilized, human chorionic gonadotropin (hCG) is secreted by the pituitary gland which increases the production of progesterone. This prevents the shedding of the endometrium as it is needed to help to nourish the developing fetus. Eventually, the production of progesterone will be taken over by the placenta. If the egg is not fertilized, the progesterone level begins to fall which leads to the shedding of the endometrium in the form of a menstrual period. The egg itself disintegrates. The low levels of estrogen and progesterone once again stimulate the hypothalamus to release GnRH, and the entire process repeats itself. The average length of a menstrual cycle is 28 days but can vary widely in length.

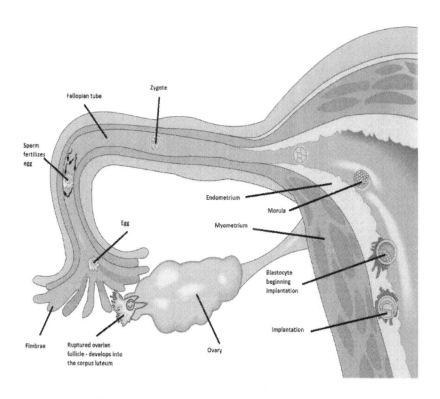

Estrogen and progesterone are in a class called steroid hormones. These hormones are built from cholesterol. Mitochondria, or small "energy centers" can be found in every living cell in our body except red blood cells. Inside the mitochondria, cholesterol is used to make a hormone called pregnenolone. From this hormone, 17-OH-pregnenolone and progesterone are synthesized. Those two hormones lead to the production of all other steroid hormones. As you can see, progesterone is essential in the synthesis of all other hormones.

According to Dr. John Lee in his book, *What Your Doctor May Not Tell You About Menopause*, "As far as we know, all of the steroid hormones are made from cholesterol. This is one of the reasons it is so important not to go on a no-fat or no-cholesterol diet" (Lee & Hopkins, 2004, p.14). This was my "ah, ha!" moment. During the seventeen years that I struggled with adenomyosis, the years that I had the most severe symptoms where in the 1990s when the no-fat diet was all the rage. I made tremendous efforts to avoid food that contained fat, and I just couldn't understand why I felt so awful. Well, now see why – my hormones were dramatically out of balance due to my no-fat diet.

Estrogen	Progesterone
Causes the endometrium to grow and thicken	Prevents further growth of the endometrium
Stimulates the breast, possibly leading to fibrocystic breast disease and/or breast cancer	Helps protect against fibrocystic breast disease and/or breast cancer
Increases blood clotting	Normalizes blood clotting
Increases body fat	Helps to use fat as an energy source
Increases risk of endometrial cancer	Protects against endometrial cancer
Causes fluid retention	Maintains water balance by acting as a diuretic
Causes insomnia and other sleep issues	Promotes normal sleep
Causes a loss of zinc and copper	Helps balance zinc and copper levels
May cause menstrual migraines	Prevents menstrual migraines
May increase anxiety and depression	Has a calming effect - helps with anxiety and depression
Interferes with blood sugar	Helps normalize blood sugar

control	levels
Little effect on sex drive	Improves sex drive
Helps prevent bone loss	Stimulates formation of new bone

As you can see from the above list, both estrogen and progesterone need to be present in the right ratio to ensure the proper functioning of the reproductive tract. It has been noted that in women with adenomyosis, the ratio of estrogen to progesterone is abnormal. There is not enough progesterone to counter the effects of estrogen. This condition is called estrogen dominance. According to Dr. John Lee and Virginia Hopkins, "Sufficient estrogen is essential to good health and is dangerous only when it is present in excess or without being balanced by progesterone and in some cases, other hormones as well" (Lee & Hopkins, p. 41). As you can see from the information above, if insufficient progesterone is produced during the luteal phase of the menstrual cycle, this could potentially cause the endometrial lining to overgrow. This overgrowth of endometrial tissue could lead to very heavy menstrual bleeding as seen in adenomyosis. In addition, we can see from the list above that too much blood clotting may take place, and this could possibly explain why women with adenomyosis tend to pass large blood clots during menstruation. Finally, the above list makes clear why these same women suffer from the well-known symptoms of PMS such as fibrocystic disease, menstrual migraines and bloating. Therefore, the subject of estrogen dominance has been addressed by so many scientists regarding its role in the development of reproductive disorders. Please see Chapter 13 for more information on this important subject.

To obtain a full understanding of hormonal balance, we need to know the function of all the major hormones. Hormones are made in the endocrine system.

The Endocrine System

The endocrine system includes tissues, organs and cells that release hormones into body fluids. The hormones produced through the endocrine system affects many metabolic processes such as water balance, blood pressure, reproduction and growth. Most hormones are either steroids, glycoproteins, amines, peptides or proteins.

The steroids are synthesized from cholesterol and include sex hormones , aldosterone and cortisol. They are soluble in fat and enter cells easily via diffusion. The amines are made in the adrenal medulla from tyrosine and include epinephrine and norepinephrine. An example of a protein hormone is parathyroid hormone. Follicle stimulating hormone (FSH) and luteinizing hormone (LH) are both glycoproteins.

Each hormone produced by the endocrine system has target cells which contain receptor sites for that specific hormone. The effects of the hormone are not activated until it binds to the receptor sites. The more receptor sites it binds to, the greater effect of the hormone.

The following chart lists organs of the endocrine system and the hormones that they secrete. In this chapter, I will specifically discuss the sex hormones. Some of the other hormones will be discussed in the next chapter.

Organs of the Endocrine System and The Hormones They Produce

Hypothalamus – Corticotropin-releasing hormone, Gonadotropin-releasing hormone (GnRH), Somatostatin, Prolactin-releasing hormone, Growth hormone-releasing hormone, Prolactin release-inhibiting hormone

Anterior pituitary gland – Adrenocorticotropic hormone, Growth hormone, Follicle-stimulating hormone (FSH), Luteinizing hormone(LH), Prolactin, Thyroid-stimulating hormone (TSH)

Posterior pituitary gland – Antidiuretic hormone, Oxytocin

Thyroid gland – Calcitonin, Thyroxin, Triiodothyronine

Parathyroid gland – Parathyroid hormone

Adrenal medulla – Epinephrine, Norepinephrine

Adrenal cortex – Aldosterone, Cortisol

Pancreas – Insulin, Glucagon, Somatostatin

Pregnenolone

I start with pregnenolone because it is the precursor to many of the other hormones discussed in this chapter. Specifically, it is a 21-carbon steroid and precursor to sex hormones and

Functions of Pregnenolone

- Precursor to estrogen, progesterone, testosterone, cortisol and DHEA
- Reduces inflammation and pain
- Improves energy
- Important in the health of the nervous system
- Improves mood
- Helps improve resistance to stress

corticosteroids. It is made from cholesterol.

Pregnenolone is synthesized by the adrenals and the central nervous system. According to University of Michigan Medicine (2018), studies have shown levels of pregnenolone are much higher in nerve tissue than in blood.

Besides being a precursor to so many important hormones, pregnenolone helps improve energy and mood. In addition, it helps to reduce inflammation and pain. Its important role of improving resistance to stress is very important for women who are struggling with adenomyosis (see Chapter 21).

Pregnenolone deficiency can be caused by a pituitary tumor, hypothyroidism or low cholesterol levels. However, supplementation should only be done under the supervision of a qualified health care practitioner.

Symptoms of a Pregnenolone Deficiency:

- Low stress tolerance
- Depression
- Fatigue
- Insomnia

Since this hormone is the precursor to so many other hormones, too much or too little of this steroid hormone could throw the entire hormonal system out of balance. Supplementation could cause problems for people who have seizures. It could also cause menstrual cycle abnormalities and could exacerbate hormone-sensitive cancers.

If, after consultation with a qualified health care practitioner, it is determined that you need pregnenolone supplementation, it is important to know the symptoms of excess pregnenolone so you are aware if you need to alter or stop supplementation. Excess pregnenolone can cause muscle aches, headaches, bloating, insomnia and racing heart.

Symptoms of an Excess of Pregnenolone:

- Headache
- Racing heart
- Muscle aches and pain
- Insomnia
- Bloating

Estrogen

This hormone has over 400 known functions in a woman's body. Some more commonly known effects include an increase in sex drive, lubrication of the vagina and its role in the menstrual cycle. However, estrogen also has effects on the body that are separate from the reproductive tract such as improving bone health, lowering LDL cholesterol, and promoting skin health.

There are several different types of estrogen, some of which are not made by the body but are found in the environment. These types are detailed below:

- **Endogenous estrogen** – estrogen made in the human body. There are several types, three of which are discussed later.

- **Phytoestrogens** – these compounds are found in plants and are generally believed to be much weaker than endogenous estrogen. Dr. John Lee and Virginia Hopkins, in their book What Doctors May Not Tell You About Menopause, state that phytoestrogens have been used to treat estrogen dominance with success (Lee & Hopkins, 2004, p. 43). However, there is some disagreement over this topic, and some recent research has shown that some phytoestrogens have estrogen activity similar to estradiol (a form of endogenous estrogen). Phytoestrogens are discussed in much more detail in Chapter 18.

- **Xenoestrogens (Xenobiotics)** – chemicals in the environment that act like estrogens in the body. The estrogen activity of these chemicals is much more potent than endogenous estrogen, so they are considered dangerous, especially in women with estrogen dominance. In addition, xenoestrogens tend to accumulate in body tissues. This topic is discussed in detail in Chapter 14.

- **Synthetic estrogens** – medications made by the pharmaceutical company that mimic the action of estrogen. The chemical alterations made in these medications make them much stronger than our endogenous estrogen. An example is birth control pills. Premarin is the most well-known form of synthetic estrogen. Since it is not chemically the same as our own estrogen, synthetics will cause side effects such as joint pain and allergies.

Major Functions of Estrogen

- Softens the cervix to allow sperm to enter the uterus and fertilize the egg
- Decreased LDL cholesterol, lipoprotein A and homocysteine levels
- Helps keep your arteries healthy by reducing plaque buildup and maintaining elasticity
- Improves sensitivity to insulin
- Reduces risk of heart disease
- Reduces risk of cataracts and macular degeneration
- Keeps your skin healthy
- Increases sex drive
- Regulates blood pressure
- Improves mood
- Lubricates vagina
- Contributes to bone health
- Helps to form neurotransmitters
- Reduces inflammation
- Increases metabolism

> *Estrogen is responsible for many of the secondary sexual characteristics in girls such as:*

- Underarm hair
- Pubic hair
- Breast enlargement
- Pigmentation of the areola
- Shape of the female body
- Development of the vagina, fallopian tubes and uterus

There are several types of endogenous estrogen. The three big ones will be discussed in this chapter: estrone (E1), estradiol (E2) and estriol (E3). E1 and E2 are produced during the reproductive years with just a very small amount of E3. During pregnancy, the major source of estrogen is E3 which is produced by the placenta. E2 is known to be the most stimulating to breast tissue, being 1,000 times more potent than estriol (Lee & Hopkins, p. 46).

- **Estrone (E1)** – Derived from estradiol (E2), this form of estrogen is the main form of estrogen after menopause. It is considered a reserve source of estrogen since it can be converted into E2. Prior to menopause, this type of estrogen is made in the ovaries, fat cells, liver and adrenal glands whereas after menopause it is made only in the fat cells. E1 is believed to increase the risk of uterine and breast cancer.

- **Estradiol (E2)** – The strongest form of estrogen, this is the main type that is produced during the reproductive years. It is twelve times stronger than E1 and eighty times stronger that E3. Estradiol is made in the ovaries and has been linked to an increase in both breast and uterine cancer.

- **Estriol (E3)** – This type of estrogen has been shown through research to have a protective effect on breast cancer. Pamela Smith, MD, MPH (2010) describes E3 as an adaptogen. This means that E3 adapts to the environment that it finds itself in and acts according to the specific needs at that time. She states "When given by itself, E3 does exert strong estrogenic effects. When given in a tenfold amount in relationship to E2, E3 antagonizes the effect of E2 and may also be another reason E3 helps decrease the risk of breast cancer".

In Chapter 13, I will discuss the topic of estrogen dominance in detail. Adenomyosis and endometriosis have been linked to a condition called estrogen dominance. This means that there is not enough progesterone in a woman's body to counter the effects of estrogen. Studies have shown that these two disorders are estrogen-dependent. Although excess estrogen is a big player in these disorders, I am going to include a list of estrogen deficiency symptoms here. If you decide to use progesterone cream (see Chapter 15 for more information), it is important to be educated on the symptoms of both progesterone excess and estrogen deficiency. If you have any of these symptoms while using progesterone cream, you may have too much progesterone in your system, and you may want to reduce or discontinue the application of the cream.

Symptoms of Estrogen Deficiency:

- Thinning hair and skin
- Infertility
- Joint pain
- Vaginal dryness
- Weight gain and inability to lose it even with proper diet and exercise
- Headaches
- Acne
- Depression and anxiety
- Oily skin
- Insomnia
- Painful intercourse
- Recurrent urinary tract infections
- Hot flashes and/or night sweats
- Fatigue
- Foggy thinking
- Low sex drive

- Bloating
- Uterine fibroids and polyps
- Moodiness, irritability, anxiety and/or depression
- Extreme fatigue
- Fibrocystic breast disease
- Periods that are heavy and prolonged
- Low sex drive

In addition, an excess of estrogen can cause hypothyroidism and increased risks of developing autoimmune disorders, endometrial cancer and breast cancer.

Progesterone

The major role of progesterone is to offset the effects of estrogen. Specifically, it inhibits the release of GnRH. Most of this hormone is made in the ovaries with lesser amounts made in the adrenal glands and some nerve cells. It is also produced in larger amounts by the corpus luteum and by the placenta during pregnancy.

During pregnancy, progesterone prevents the uterus from contracting in order to maintain the pregnancy. Progesterone levels in pregnancy are about ten times higher than in non-pregnant women.

Progesterone can decrease the amount of time E2 stays in its receptor site which will result in lower levels of estrogen in a woman's body. In addition, progesterone may decrease the strength and frequency of uterine contractions in both adenomyosis and endometriosis. This hormone also helps with insomnia, has calming effects, regulates blood sugar levels and increases sex drive.

Functions of Progesterone:

- Improves memory
- Increases sex drive
- Helps to balance blood sugar levels
- Helps build bone
- Has a calming effect – reduces anxiety and mood swings
- Promotes healthy sleep patterns
- Improves digestion

A woman's body produces about 20-30 mg of progesterone a day during the luteal phase of the menstrual cycle. In addition to its role in offsetting the effects of estrogen, progesterone is Also involved in the production of new bone, so it plays an important role in preventing osteoporosis.

According to Pamela Smith, M.D., MPH (2010), "high progesterone levels can only result if a woman is taking too much progesterone or too much pregnenolone."

- Increase in appetite
- Increase in carbohydrate cravings
- Increases insulin levels which may lead to insulin resistance
- May cause incontinence
- May suppress the immune system
- Decreases the level of growth hormone
- Increases the level of cortisol

Follicle Stimulating Hormone (FSH) and Luteinizing Hormone (LH)

FSH and LH are glycoproteins and are members of the hormone group called gonadotropins. Gonadotropins stimulate the ovaries and are essential for reproduction. FSH is responsible for the growth of the ovarian follicles that contain the eggs, and it also stimulates the production of estrogen. LH is responsible for the release of the egg from the mature ovarian follicle and for the growth of the corpus luteum. The hypothalamus secretes gonadotropin-releasing hormone, or GnRH, which stimulates the production of both FSH and LH. These two hormones are secreted from the anterior pituitary gland.

Increased levels of FSH may indicate menopause or primary ovarian failure. Increased levels of LH may be a sign of menopause, primary ovarian failure or polycystic ovarian syndrome (PCOS). Low levels of FSH may indicate PCOS, and low levels of either FSH or LH may occur in primary ovarian hyperfunction.

Androgens

Androgens are a class of hormones that are responsible for male characteristics; however, these hormones are also present in women in small amounts, and they serve important functions in the female body. Testosterone and androstenedione are two types of androgens. In addition, for E2 to function optimally, testosterone levels must be present in optimal levels.

Testosterone

A member of the androgens, testosterone does have functions in the female. It maintains a healthy sex drive and helps maintain muscle and bone growth.

This hormone is made in the ovaries and adrenal glands. Interestingly, only one percent of the testosterone in a woman's body is "free". This means that only one percent is available for the body to use. The rest of the hormone is bound to a substance called sex-hormone binding globulin, also called SHBG. This substance is made in the liver and to lesser amounts in the brain, vagina, uterus and placenta. If SHBG levels are low, then the levels of both "free" E2 and testosterone increase. The reverse is also true. If SHBG levels are high, then the levels of "free" E2 and testosterone decrease. Low SHBG levels may indicate hypothyroidism, polycystic ovarian syndrome and diabetes. High

SHBG levels may indicate hyperthyroidism, anorexia and pregnancy.

Functions of Testosterone

- Increases muscle mass and tone
- Decreases body fat
- Improves bone health
- Increases sex drive
- Improves ability to focus
- Improves memory
- Helps to prevent bone loss
- Supports the production of neurotransmitters which results in improved mood.

A connection between the levels of SHBG, insulin and prolactin levels has been described in the literature. A study by Plymate, Matei, Jones and Freidl showed that SHBG levels were decreased in the presence of high insulin and prolactin levels in a human hepatoma cell line. They concluded that "insulin and [prolactin] inhibit SHBG production...". This again reinforces the role of all hormones in hormonal balance.

A testosterone deficiency has been seen in women who are in menopause, who have endometriosis, who are on birth control pills and who are under stress.

Symptoms of a Testosterone Deficiency

- Low sex drive
- Decrease in muscle tone and strength
- Fatigue
- Depression
- Anxiety
- Weight gain
- Decrease in HDL cholesterol (good cholesterol)
- Loss of skin elasticity
- Memory problems
- Bone loss
- Dry and thinning hair

If you find that you have a testosterone deficiency through hormonal testing, it can be treated successfully with a natural testosterone cream. It is of utmost importance to alternate the location of the application of the cream. If you apply it to the same location repeatedly, excess hair growth in that area may result. It is also important to avoid synthetic testosterone as it has been linked to liver cancer.

One of the most common hormonal disorders in women is high testosterone. This hormonal imbalance causes excess body hair, weight gain, mood swings, and anger outbursts.

Symptoms of High Testosterone

- Excess body hair including hirsutism (excess facial hair)
- Problems in anger control
- Acne
- Oily skin
- Bloating
- Fatigue
- Mood swings/depression
- Weight gain
- Infertility
- Irregular menstrual cycles

According to Lee and Hopkins (2006), Dr. David Zava has seen women where their androgen levels were normal to high, but their libido was low. These women were found to either have estrogen dominance or were under high stress levels. This emphasized the point that all the hormones must be in balance for optimum health.

DHEA

Also known as dehydroepiandrosterone, DHEA is another important androgen that is needed for the proper functioning of the entire hormonal system in a woman's body. Specifically, it helps a woman deal more effectively with stress. It is the precursor to the estrogens and testosterone and is important in protein building. It is made predominately in the adrenal glands. According to Pamela Smith, M.D., M.P.H., (2010), "by the age of seventy, your body only makes one-fourth of the amount it made [in your twenties]."

Note: Only use DHEA under the supervision of a physician. Not enough is known about this supplement and how it affects hormone levels. Much more research needs to be done.

Functions of DHEA

- Lowers triglycerides and cholesterol
- Supports the immune system
- Helps to control blood sugar levels
- May help to improve mood and fatigue
- Decreases allergies
- Improves bone health
- May help to reduce body fat
- Helps to reduce stress levels
- Helps to maintain a healthy weight
- May help with infertility

According to Pamela Smith, MD, MPH (2010), DHEA has been shown to "have a protective effect against cancer, diabetes, obesity, high cholesterol, heart disease and autoimmune diseases."

Symptoms of a DHEA Deficiency

1. Lack of energy
2. Weight gain
3. Joint soreness
4. Decrease in muscle mass and strength
5. High stress levels

Symptoms of DHEA Excess

- Irritability and mood swings
- Weight gain
- Fatigue
- Depression
- Anger issues/lack of temper control
- Hirsutism (facial hair)
- Insomnia
- Acne

Again, DHEA supplementation should only be done under the supervision of a qualified health care practitioner. Taking a DHEA supplement may help with depression, osteoporosis and vaginal atrophy in postmenopausal women. In addition, it may help to slow the aging process. However, since DHEA is a hormone, it may worsen mood disorders, cause excess hair growth on the body and cause oily skin and acne. It is contraindicated for use in cases of hormone-sensitive disorders, pregnancy and breast feeding.

If you and your physician decide it might help you to try DHEA, it is important to know that the body cannot make DHEA from a wild yam extract. If the supplement says that it is a "wild yam extract", don't bother buying it. It won't do a thing. The supplement must be actual DHEA to be effective. If you aren't sure about a supplement, call the manufacturer.

Chapter 3 - Other Important Hormones

"All the hormones in your body interact with each other. They are a web; a symphony that must play in tune in order for you to feel great and be healthy."

-Pamela Wartian Smith from her book, What You Must Know About Women's Hormones

In addition to the sex hormones that were covered in the previous chapter, the following hormones are also extremely important in the proper functioning of the reproductive tract. All these hormones interact with each other and affect their levels. It is important to realize this as you try and achieve proper hormone balance in attempt to control the symptoms of adenomyosis.

Cortisol

Cortisol is a glucocorticoid that is produced in the adrenal cortex. This hormone affects glucose, protein and fat metabolism. Most people know that cortisol levels are linked to stress. However, cortisol is very important to the health of your immune system.

When your stress level is high, cortisol levels are high. Since this hormone is made in the adrenal glands, it is important to keep your adrenal glands healthy. If the adrenals are fatigued, levels of both cortisol and DHEA drop which obviously will lead to a hormonal imbalance. See more about the effects of stress on hormonal balance in Chapter 21.

When your adrenals are fatigued and cortisol levels become deficient, you may feel tired all the time. In addition, you may have sugar cravings, need afternoon naps, be unable to lose weight, have chemical sensitivities and/or allergies, or may be unable to sleep through the night.

Functions of Cortisol

1. Helps to deal with stress
2. Influences the ratio of estrogen to testosterone
3. Influences the ratio of DHEA to insulin
4. Improves sleep quality
5. Helps to keep blood sugar levels balanced
6. Improves mood
7. Helps with weight control

Conditions Associated with Abnormal Levels of Cortisol:

1. Chronic fatigue syndrome
2. Fibromyalgia
3. Premenstrual syndrome
4. Depression
5. Insomnia and other sleep disorders
6. Infertility

Supplementation with DHEA may help with adrenal fatigue and low cortisol levels. However, DHEA may also increase estrogen levels, so supplementation with this hormone is only advised under the supervision of a health care practitioner. Other nutrients that may aid in adrenal support include the B vitamins, vitamin C, calcium, magnesium, copper, zinc and omega-3 fatty acids.

In addition to the above nutrients, the following list contains additional lifestyle changes that may help support the adrenals:

- Stress reduction if possible
- Getting a full night of sleep (8 hours if possible)
- Meditation for stress reduction
- Massage for stress reduction
- Exercise to help deal more effectively with stress (tai chi and yoga are good options)

Insulin

Most people know that insulin helps to regulate your blood sugar levels. It is a hormone that is produced in the beta cells of the pancreas. When glucose levels rise as a result of eating food high in sugar, insulin is released from the beta cells. It is the job of insulin to move glucose out of the bloodstream and into cells. This action reduces the level of blood glucose which keeps these levels in check. Insulin also promotes the movement of amino acids into cells and stimulates fat tissue to manufacture and store fat. When glucose levels are low, the beta cells inhibit the secretion of insulin.

In a person with diabetes, the beta cells are either destroyed (Type 1) or work less efficiently (Type II). Therefore, insulin in diabetics is either not produced or produced less efficiently, hence the need for insulin in these patients.

Functions of Insulin

- Promotes the production of serotonin
- Counteracts the action of adrenaline
- Converts blood sugar into triglycerides
- Counteracts the action of cortisol

Insulin resistance is a term used to describe a condition where the body poorly responds or does not respond at all to insulin. This occurs when a person has a diet consistently high in sugar. In the insulin receptor, there is an enzyme called tyrosine kinase. When insulin locks into the receptor, tyrosine kinase is activated and allows glucose to enter cells. In insulin resistance, tyrosine kinase fails to do its job. Because the body does not respond to insulin in this condition, more insulin is produced. This prolonged elevation in insulin levels causes the theca cells in the adrenal glands to produce an enzyme called 17,20-lyase which tells your body to stop making estrogen and to make androgens instead. Again, this demonstrates how insulin can play a role in hormonal balance in the reproductive tract.

Causes of Insulin Resistance

- Diet high is processed food
- Diet high in sugar
- Missing meals
- Stress
- Environmental toxins

Causes of High Insulin

- Eating a diet high in sugar
- Frequent consumption of soft drinks
- A low-fat diet
- High intake of caffeine
- Consumption of artificial sweeteners
- Lack of exercise
- Medications including birth control pills, steroids, thiazide diuretics, beta-blockers and medications that contain caffeine (such as pain relievers or cold medications)

Foods that Adversely Affect Insulin Levels

- Processed sugar
- White rice
- White potatoes
- Products that contain white flour
- Processed food

To keep insulin levels in check, eat a balanced diet and exercise at least three times a week. Pamela Smith, MD, MPH (2010) also suggests the use of alpha lipoic acid, chromium and vitamin D. However, she also urges those who are diabetic to closely monitor their blood sugar levels if supplementing with these nutrients. It is advisable to consult with your health care practitioner about these supplements before taking them if you are diabetic.

Thyroid Hormone

Thyroid hormone levels are extremely important in women's health. According to the website yourhormonebalance.com in an article titled *How Hormones Work* (2018), "women have an approximately seven times greater risk for developing thyroid problems than do men." They also state "some 26 percent of women in or near menopause are diagnosed with hypothyroidism."

The following are the types of thyroid hormones:

- TSH – thyroid stimulating hormone – a glycoprotein, also known as thyrotropin
- T2 - diiodothyronine
- T3 – triiodothyronine
- T4 – Thyroxine – also known as tetraiodothyronine.

Iodine is vital to produce thyroid hormones along with the amino acid tyrosine.

TSH is made in the pituitary gland and is partially regulated by the hypothalamus. T2 increases the metabolic rate in muscles and fat. T3 is five times as active as T4. Eighty percent of the production of the thyroid gland is T4, and most of it is converted into the more active T3 in the liver and/or kidneys.

T4 can also be changed into reverse T3 which is an inactive form of T3. Reverse T3 is only 1% as active of T3, and it occupies the same receptor site, so if reverse T3 levels are high, thyroid hormone levels may be decreased – a condition known as hypothyroidism. One of the main causes of an elevation in reverse T3 is stress since chronically high cortisol levels lead to the production of more reverse T3. According to Pamela Smith (2010), other causes of reverse T3 include autoimmune disease, nutritional deficiencies, environmental toxins, electromagnetic radiation, infections, unhealthy liver and hormonal imbalances.

Functions of the Thyroid Gland:

- Regulates hormones
- Controls blood flow
- Controls use of vitamins and the metabolism of proteins, carbohydrates and fats
- Regulates sexual function
- Controls energy production and utilization
- Controls the action of muscles and nerves

Symptoms of Hypothyroidism

- Dry hair and skin
- Constipation
- Fatigue
- Weight gain
- Low blood pressure
- High cholesterol

According to Pamela Smith (2010), hypothyroidism can cause "an increase in production of hydroxyestrone. It can also lead to a decrease in SHBG which increases the bioavailable amount of E2 and testosterone in the body." Again, this shows how thyroid hormone levels can impact the activity of sex hormones.

The enzyme 5'diodinase is needed for the proper conversion of T4 to T3. Factors such as chronic illness, liver or kidney dysfunction, excess levels of estrogen, stress, birth control pills, a diet high in carbohydrates and low in protein, pesticides and herbicides have all been implicated in decreased levels of 5'diodinase. In addition, the following are known to play a role in decreased levels of T3 due to improper conversion from T4:

- Not enough adrenal hormones such as DHEA
- Phthalates
- Dioxins
- PCBs
- Excess calcium
- Excess copper
- Lead
- Mercury
- Fluoride

The following nutrients have been shown to be helpful in the conversion of T4 to T3:

- Selenium
- Zinc
- Vitamin D
- Iron
- Iodine
- Vitamins B6 and B12
- Melatonin

Hyperthyroidism can also cause irregular menstruation. In addition, it causes intolerance to heat, nervousness, a rapid

---

Symptoms of Hyperthyroidism

---

1. Weight loss
2. Intolerance to heat
3. Excessive sweating
4. Insomnia
5. Anxiety, irritability

---

heart rate and protruding eyeballs. This condition occurs when too much thyroxine is produced.

Causes of hyperthyroidism include Graves disease, and thyroiditis. Graves disease is an autoimmune disorder that causes the body to produce too much T4. Thyroiditis is an inflammation of the thyroid gland. This inflammation causes the glad to store excess thyroid hormone, and some of the excess leaks out into the bloodstream causing the hormone levels to increase.

Thyroid medications, radioactive iodine and surgery to remove all or part of the thyroid gland are all effective treatments for hyperthyroidism.

Melatonin

Made from the amino acid tryptophan, melatonin is responsible to regulating your wake/sleep cycle. It is made in the pineal gland which responds to nerve impulses from the retina of the eye. If there is light, the pineal gland will secrete less melatonin, whereas if there is darkness, the pineal gland will secrete more melatonin.

Functions of Melatonin

- Antioxidant
- Improves mood
- Improves sleep quality
- Stimulates the production of growth hormone
- Decreases cortisol
- Involved in the release of sex hormones
- Increases the activity of the immune system

Excess melatonin may lead to a suppression of estrogen and testosterone production. A deficiency of estrogen can suppress the release of growth hormone which may lead to premature aging. However, According to Pamela Smith (2010), melatonin blocks estrogen from binding to its receptors. In women who are suffering from adenomyosis and estrogen dominance, increasing melatonin production may actually help; however, keep in mind that excess melatonin may also lead to other problems. It is advisable to work with a health care practitioner when trying to achieve hormone balance.

Prolactin

Prolactin is a protein hormone produced in the pituitary gland and is responsible for milk production after childbirth. The hypothalamus regulates its release. Levels of prolactin increase and stimulate the mammary glands right after childbirth in preparation for breast feeding.

Prolactin is known to suppress the actions of dopamine and GnRH. The suppression of GnRH leads to low FSH and LH levels which causes disruptions in the normal menstrual cycle. Excess levels of prolactin are known to reduce estrogen levels in women.

Low prolactin levels reduce milk production after childbirth. Women that have problems breast feeding due to lack of milk may be deficient in prolactin.

Symptoms of High Prolactin Levels

- Depression
- Infertility
- Discharge from the breast
- Engorged breasts
- Breast tenderness
- Menstrual abnormalities
- Weight gain
- Bone loss

High prolactin levels (hyperprolactinemia) have been noted in women with adenomyosis. However, many more studies need to be done to determine the significance of this finding.

Causes of High Prolactin Levels

- Pituitary tumor called a prolactinoma
- Hypothyroidism
- Disorders of the hypothalamus
- Stress
- Medications

Chapter 4 - Liver Detoxification

"A body with a healthy immune system, efficient organs of elimination and detoxification, and a sound circulatory and nervous system can handle a great deal of toxicity."

-Dr. Leon Chaitow

As you will see later in this book, detoxification and liver health are extremely important in hormone balance. Specifically, since adenomyosis is an estrogen-dependent disorder, it is imperative to keep the liver functioning properly so it can break down and eliminate estrogen from the body effectively. Understanding how liver detoxification occurs will help the reader understand why certain supplements are important in the diet (see Chapter 20).

Detoxification is the process in which toxic substances are eliminated from the body. These toxins include medications, environmental pollutants and byproducts of metabolism such as estrogen metabolites. The detoxification process occurs through the skin (sweat), kidneys (urine), gastrointestinal tract (stool) and the liver. A healthy liver is extremely important in this detoxification process.

A vital organ, the liver is located in the upper right quadrant of the abdomen and has many important functions. It stores vitamins and minerals, makes blood clotting factors, stores glycogen which can be converted into glucose for energy, breaks down nutrients and is heavily involved in detoxification of toxins that enter the body. These toxins are broken down by Kupffer cells in the liver. The liver also produces bile which is required for the digestion of fats. Of utmost importance in the discussion of adenomyosis is the breakdown and elimination of estrogen. Since estrogen is metabolized in the liver, it is necessary to keep the liver healthy to keep estrogen levels in check. The liver follows three detoxification pathways – Phase I, Phase II and Phase III.

Phase I (Modification)

In Phase I, the liver converts dangerous toxins into metabolites through the use of enzymes. These toxins are the end-products of metabolism, drugs, chemicals, pollutants and microbial endotoxins. Fifty to 100 cytochrome P450 enzymes are used during this phase. There are five chemical reactions that occur during phase I:

- Oxidation
- Reduction
- Hydrolysis
- Hydration
- Dehalogenation

These reactions transform dangerous toxins to less harmful substances that can be metabolized during Phase II. However, in converting these toxins into less harmful substances, free radicals are formed, and these can potentially damage liver cells. The liver produces glutathione which is an antioxidant. If the liver is functioning optimally, it produces enough glutathione to neutralize the free radicals produced through the Phase I process. However, if the liver isn't functioning properly, not enough glutathione is produced which may not only lead to liver damage but will also reduce the ability of the liver to break down toxins. In addition, if the Phase I process isn't working efficiently, these toxic substances may not be properly broken down which will result in the buildup of toxins, including estrogen.

The nutrients that promote proper functioning of this pathway include vitamin A, vitamin B2, vitamin B3, vitamin B6, vitamin B12, vitamin C, vitamin D3, vitamin E, calcium, bioflavonoids, N-acetyl cysteine, quercetin, lipoic acid, grape seed extract, glutathione, copper, folic acid, magnesium and zinc. In addition, the following herbs are excellent to add to the diet in order to optimize liver detoxification: cascara sagrada (use sparingly), chia, coenzyme Q10, dandelion, lemon balm, marshmallow, milk thistle, mullein, pycnogenol, psyllium fiber, senna (use sparingly) and slippery elm. More detailed information on these herbs can be found in Chapter 20.

Phase II (Conjugation)

In Phase II, the metabolites formed from Phase I bind to another substance (cysteine, glycine or sulfur) which neutralizes the toxin. This is done by converting the toxin from a fat-soluble substance to a water-soluble substance. This process is accomplished in six steps:

- Glutathione conjugation
- Amino acid conjugation
- Methylation
- Sulfation
- Acetylation
- Glucuronidation

Nutrients that aid in the proper functioning of the Phase II pathway include taurine, methionine, folic acid, calcium d-glucarate, sulfur, indole-3-carbinol, N-acetyl cysteine, choline and inositol.

Phase III (Excretion)

Phase III further metabolizes the conjugates from Phase II through the antiporter system. More than 350 antiporter proteins are concentrated in the small intestine and are responsible for the transport of the metabolites out of the hepatocytes (liver cells) via the efflux pump. The most well-known antiporter protein is P-glycoprotein. This step requires energy in the form of ATP.

Nutrients necessary for the optimal functioning of Phase III include fiber, adequate water intake, B vitamins, coenzyme Q10, magnesium, polyphenols and sulforaphane. Apples are an excellent source of polyphenols and broccoli is a great source of sulforaphane.

It is necessary to keep all phases of the liver detoxification pathways functioning optimally to encourage proper neutralization and elimination of estrogen. It is important to know, however, that there are both "good" estrogen metabolites and "bad" estrogen metabolites. The metabolites 2-(OH)-estrone and 2-(OH)-estradiol are considered good metabolites as they are known to be strong antioxidants. The levels of these good estrogens are usually seen in women who exercise moderately and eat a high protein/low-fat diet. They also lower LDL (bad) cholesterol and raise HDL (good) cholesterol. The metabolites 16 alpha-(OH)-estrone and 4-(OH)-estrone are "bad" estrogen metabolites. In particular, 16 alpha-(OH)-estrone has been shown to be even more powerful than estradiol (Lam, 2015b). These toxic substances have also been linked to breast cancer and have a powerful effect on estrogen receptor sites.

As I'm sure you've already concluded, a healthy diet full of vitamins and minerals is necessary to keep the liver functioning properly. Supplements may also be a good idea, especially if your diet is lacking in fresh, organic fruits and vegetables. Bitter herbs have the amazing ability to aid in digestion and have a beneficial effect on the proper functioning of the liver. These herbs are listed below, and it would be wise to incorporate them into the diet to keep the liver functioning at an optimal level. To learn more about the following herbs, please see Chapter 20.

- Cascara Sagrada
- Chia
- Dandelion
- Lemon Balm
- Marshmallow
- Milk Thistle
- Mullein
- Psyllium fiber

- Senna
- Slippery Elm

By keeping the liver functioning properly, it will be better able to process dangerous toxins, especially the dangerous xenoestrogens that may be a contributor to adenomyosis development. A healthy liver will also be able to process estrogen efficiently which will aid in proper elimination, reducing the chance of developing estrogen dominance.

Chapter 5 - Eicosanoids

"Symptoms, then are in reality nothing but the cry from suffering organs."

-Jean Martin Charcot (translated from French)

As you will learn later, omega-3 fatty acids play a huge role in reducing inflammation in the body. They have also been shown to be possibly useful in the treatment of adenomyosis and endometriosis. This chapter will explain how eicosanoids function in the inflammatory processes in the body.

Eicosanoids are a type of hormone that requires polyunsaturated fat for their synthesis and have over one hundred known functions. These substances have both helpful and harmful effects in the body, so it is important that they are present in a balanced ratio. "Good" eicosanoids prevent blood clots, dilate blood vessels, reduce pain, enhance the immune system and improve brain function. "Bad" eicosanoids promote blood clots, constrict blood vessels, promote pain and decrease immune and brain function. Balance of these hormones are imperative for optimum health. For example, the eicosanoid which decreases blood clotting counteracts the one that stimulates the clotting. The stimulation of blood clotting is important when someone is bleeding as the eicosanoid will help to stop the bleeding; however, if the blood clots too much, this can lead to possible cardiovascular disease or stroke.

Other known functions of eicosanoids include regulation of blood pressure, control of allergic responses and regulation of smooth muscle contraction. The different groups of eicosanoids include the prostaglandins (PG) which regulate pain and inflammation, prostacyclins (PGI) which decrease blood clotting, thromboxanes (TX) which stimulate blood clotting, leukotrienes (LT) which control the inflammatory response, and lipoxins (LX) which play a role in immune and allergic responses. An increase in "bad" eicosanoids causes inflammation through proteins produced by immune cells called cytokines. These cytokines can lead to the production of more "bad" eicosanoids, and a vicious cycle starts. According to Barry Sears, "eicosanoid control has 90% of the impact on the pain you feel."

As previously mentioned, both omega-3 and omega-6 fatty acids are precursors to prostaglandins. Prostaglandins are a type of eicosanoid which regulate pain, inflammation and swelling. They play a role in digestion, blood pressure control, heart function, kidney function, allergic reactions, blood clotting and hormone production. Omega-3 fatty acids make certain kinds of prostaglandins while omega-6 fatty acids make other kinds. Alpha-linolenic acid (LNA) and eicosapentenoic acid (EPA) are both omega-3 fatty acids They produce the "good" eicosanoids, also referred to as the series I eicosanoids. EPA also leads to the production of series III eicosanoids, another group of "good" eicosanoids. Linoleic acid (LA), an omega-6 fatty acid, produces the "bad" eicosanoids, or the series II eicosanoids. Arachidonic acid is an example of a "bad" eicosanoid that is produced by LA.

"Good" eicosanoids can also be produced through the LA (omega-6) pathway through the action of dihomogamma linolenic acid (DGLA) as seen in the reaction below. DGLA leads to the production of both series I and series II eicosanoids.

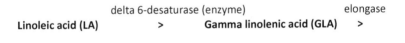

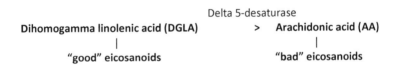

The balance of DGLA and AA will determine what kind of eicosanoid will be produced. An example of a "good" eicosanoid produced from DGLA is the prostaglandin PGE1. This prostaglandin is a good vasodilator, inhibitor of platelet aggregation and a reducer of insulin secretion. Another powerful eicosanoid produced from DGLA is PGA1. This is a strong suppressor of viral replication, and it inhibits NF kappa B which reduces inflammation by suppressing the production of pro-inflammatory cytokines. DGLA also leads to the production of 15-HETriE which is a potent inhibitor of leukotriene synthesis.

High levels of insulin activate delta 5-desaturase which leads to the production of more AA and "bad" eicosanoids. Remember that high insulin levels are predominately a result of a high-sugar diet. AA promotes an increased release of pro-inflammatory cytokines. AA also produces the prostaglandin PGE2 and the leukotriene LTB4, both of which promote inflammation. Other "bad" eicosanoids produced through the AA pathway include the lipoxins A4 and B4 and the prostacyclin PG12. In addition, AA produces TXA2 which decreases blood flow.

The following is a list of some of the pro-inflammatory eicosanoids and a short description of their function:

1. **Prostaglandin E2 (PGE2)** – induces fever, stimulates uterine contractions during childbirth.

2. **Leukotriene B4 (LTB4)** – produced by leukocytes and causes inflammation.

3. **Prostaglandin D2 (PGD2)** – produced by mast cells and is active in allergic responses and asthma.

4. **Thromboxane A2 (TXA2)** – stimulates the activation of new platelets and promotes clotting.

5. **Leukotriene C4 (LTC4)** – promotes allergic responses and asthma, active during liver injury, cardiovascular disease, atherosclerosis and colon cancer.

6. **Leukotriene D4 (LTD4)** – involved in the constriction of smooth muscle such as bronchoconstriction and vasoconstriction. Active in asthma.

7. **Hydroxyeicosatetraenoic acids (HETEs) and oxoeicosanoids (oxo-ETEs)** – these eicosanoids send leukocytes and macrophages (white blood cells that fight infection) to the site of tissue injury which results in inflammation.

The following is a list of the anti-inflammatory eicosanoids and a short description of their function:

1. **15-deoxy-delta(12,14)-prostaglandin J2 (15-d-Δ12,14-PGJ2)** – potent anti-inflammatory that is active in repressing inflammation in endotoxic shock according to a study by Kaplan et al. (2005).

2. **Lipoxin A4 and B4 (LxA4 and LxB4)** – both stimulate anti-inflammatory pathways which reduces and resolves inflammation. They are members of SPMs (specialized pro-resolving mediators) which are involved in tissue healing and protection.

3. **Resolvin E1 and E2 (RvE1 and RvE2)** – potent anti-inflammatories that are members of the SPMs. According to Wikipedia (2017), "[Resolvins] failure to form in adequate amounts is also proposed to underlie a broad range of human diseases involving pathological inflammation."

4. **14,15-EET** – a type of epoxyeicosatetrionic acid that has antihypertensive and anti-inflammatory properties. Although they are short-lived, they stimulate vasorelaxation.

EPA (omega-3) is converted into the series II eicosanoids which have been shown to lower triglycerides, reduce pain and inflammation from rheumatoid arthritis and inhibit the production of AA. The pathway in which LNA is converted into EPA is shown below:

	Delta-6 desaturase		elongase	
Alpha linolenic acid (LNA)	>	**Steradonic acid**	>	

	Delta-5 desaturase		elongase x 2	
Eicosatretaconic acid	>	**Eicosapentenoic acid (EPA)**	>	

	Delta-6 desaturase		peroxisomal oxidation	
24-long carbon chain, 5 double bonds	>	**24-long carbon chain, 6 double bonds**	>	

	Peroxisomal oxidation	
Docosahexanoic acid (DHA)	>	**eicosapentenoic acid (EPA)** – see above Process is repeated to produce more DHA

EPA inhibits the production of AA thereby reducing the production of "bad" eicosanoids. EPA also inhibits the delta 5-desaturase enzyme which promotes a more balanced ratio of DGLA to AA in the LA pathway.

Proper balance of both the good eicosanoids and the bad eicosanoids is essential for optimum health. The following chart details some of the ways the balance of eicosanoids could shift:

Ways in Which the Balance of Eicosanoids Can Shift

- High insulin shifts the balance toward the "bad" eicosanoids.
- Trans-fatty acids shift the balance toward the "bad" eicosanoids.
- Glucagon, a hormone released from the pancreas that increases blood sugar levels, shifts the balance toward the "good" eicosanoids.
- LNA (flaxseed/ fish oil), EPA and DHA (fish) shift the balance toward the "good" eicosanoids.

Once fatty acids are released from cell membranes through the action of phospholipase A2, they follow one of three pathways:

1. Cyclo-oxygenase pathway (COX)
2. 5-lipoxygenase pathway
3. 12 or 15-lipoxygenase pathway

The COX pathway produces thromboxanes and prostaglandins. There are two types of COX enzymes in this pathway: COX 1 and COX 2. COX 1 enzymes are in vascular cells that line the bloodstream and stomach, and they secrete bicarbonate which neutralizes stomach acid. The COX-2 enzyme is release in response to inflammation.

The 5-lipoxygenase pathway, also known as 5-LIPO, leads to the production of leukotrienes.

The 12 or 15-lipoxygenase pathway leads to the production of hydroxylated fatty acids and lipoxins.

There are very few inhibitors of the LIPO enzymes. Corticosteroids work but have many side effects. In addition, cortisol, released from the adrenal glands as a result of stress, synthesizes lipocortin which inhibits the action of phospholipase A2 in an attempt to stop the production of "bad" eicosanoids. This may sound good, but as I previously stated, phospholipase A2 is necessary for fatty acids to be released from the cell membranes. In short, excess cortisol reduces the amounts of fatty acids that the body can use. This can depress the immune system, disrupt short-term memory and destroy nerve cells in the brain in addition to causing an increase in inflammation.

Section II

Chapter 6 - Adenomyosis and Endometriosis – What is the Difference?

"Anyone can fake being sick, but it takes a really strong woman to fake being well."

-Jill Fuersich

Adenomyosis and endometriosis are sometimes discussed together. There is good reason for that. At one time, adenomyosis was referred to as "endometriosis interna". That has now changed, but it does indicate some similarity between the two disorders. While adenomyosis refers to endometrial-like tissue that has invaded the uterine muscle (myometrium), endometriosis refers to endometrial-like tissue that is present outside of the uterus. These endometrial-like implants can be found on the bladder, bowel, ovaries, lungs and many other locations throughout the female body. In fact, there has been a case of endometriosis in a male. To complicate the matter even further, the symptoms of adenomyosis and endometriosis are similar.

In many cases, adenomyosis and endometriosis occur together. Kunz et al. (2007) state adenomyosis and endometriosis may be different forms of the same disease since both involve displaced endometrial-like tissue. In addition, these same investigators determined that in a group of women with known endometriosis, 70% also had adenomyosis as compared to a normal control group in which only 9% of women were found to have the disorder. Although this same group of researchers found a significantly higher rate of adenomyosis in women with endometriosis, Bazot et al. (2001) only found 27% of women with endometriosis also had adenomyosis. The discrepancy can be blamed on the different imaging criteria that are currently being used to diagnose the disorders. Dr. Albee at the Center for Endometriosis Care (2017) states, "In my experience at the Center for Endometriosis Care, every time a patient has requested hysterectomy after conservative surgery for endometriosis failed to control severe dysmenorrhea (cramps) or central pelvic pain, adenomyosis has been found in the uterus."

In addition, a 2006 study showed that in women who had excision of endometriosis but who continued to have pelvic pain after surgery had a thickened junctional zone of >11 mm on MRI imaging prior to surgery. This continuing pelvic pain and thickened junctional zone may indicate the presence of adenomyosis.

An interesting study done by Millischer et al. (2013) showed the presence of adenomyosis could be a marker of deep intestinal endometriosis. They found 76% of patients with diffuse adenomyosis had more than one deep intestinal lesion as compared to the control group without adenomyosis. Also, if the adenomyosis was focal and located in the posterior section of the uterus, the number of intestinal lesions was greater. Eighty-seven percent of those with focal adenomyosis in the posterior section of the uterus had three or more intestinal lesions.

According to the EFA (2015), endometriosis can be easily misdiagnosed as adenomyosis, appendicitis, bowel obstruction, colon cancer, diverticulitis, ectopic pregnancy, fibroids, inflammatory bowel disease, irritable bowel syndrome, ovarian cancer, ovarian cysts and pelvic inflammatory disease. Because this disorder can be so easily misdiagnosed, it is imperative that the patient who experiences any of the above symptoms be seen by an expert in the field of endometriosis and adenomyosis.

The following chart gives some interesting basic facts about endometriosis. These facts were obtained from the Endometriosis Foundation of America. The one that personally interests me the most is how endometriosis is commonly misdiagnosed as IBS. I had that diagnosis all the way until my hysterectomy – 17 years!!

> ## The following are some interesting facts on endometriosis (EFA, 2015):

- On average, it takes a woman ten years to obtain a correct diagnosis of endometriosis.
- Approximately 176 million women suffer from this disorder worldwide.
- Bowel symptoms of endometriosis are commonly misdiagnosed as irritable bowel syndrome (IBS).
- Endometriosis is commonly misdiagnosed as pelvic inflammatory disease (PID).
- Cost of the disorder are estimated to be about $22 billion annually.
- Endometriosis is one of the top three causes of female infertility.

An interesting fact about endometriosis is that pain level does not correlate with the amount of endometriosis present. Some women with very little endometriosis may suffer from debilitating pain while other women with severe endometriosis may have very little pain. It is important to know the amount of pain present does not indicate the severity of the disease. It is also important to note that the tissue of endometriosis is endometrial-like, but it is not identical to the tissue of the endometrium. According to the Endometriosis Foundation of America (EFA, 2015), endometriosis has been associated with autoimmune disease. However, there really is no consensus on what causes this disorder. It has been noted that a woman is seven times more likely to have endometriosis if her mother suffered from it (EFA, 2015).

Endometriosis can affect the lungs, diaphragm and sciatic region of the back. This disorder has been known to cause a collapsed lung when it involved the pleural cavity.

Possible risk factors for the development of endometriosis

- Estrogen dominance
- Poor diet
- Dysfunction of the immune system – IL-8, TNF-alpha and IL-10 have been noted to be increased in women with endometriosis, and women with endometriosis have a higher than normal rate of other autoimmune diseases.
- Menstrual cycles that occur more often than every 28 days
- Exposure to xenoestrogens (man-made chemicals that act like estrogen in the body)
- Poor liver health

According to Pamela Smith (2010), in a study of more than 500 women, "there was a 40 percent decreased risk of developing endometriosis in those who ate more green vegetables and fresh fruit...there was an 80 percent increase in risk of developing endometriosis in those who ate large amounts of red meat. This emphasizes the importance of a healthy diet in dealing with this disorder.

Rare Cases of Endometriosis in Men

The following is a copy of a blog that I wrote on Adenomyosis Fighters in 2016. I include it here as I found it quite interesting that there have been documented cases of endometriosis in men. This information may eventually give even more insight to the pathogenesis of this disorder.

Yes, you read that right! There are a few rare cases of endometriosis that have been found in men. I read an article the other day that addressed this issue, and I was shocked! Before I wrote this blog, however, I wanted to verify that this is true. Well, it is. It's rare, but it has happened.

A study published in 1985 by Martin and Hauck looked at an 83-year-old man who had an endometrioma on his lower abdominal wall. The researchers reference several other cases that have been reported in the literature. The theory for the development of endometriosis-like tissue in the male at that time was that it developed from remnants of the prostatic utricle, or remnants of the uterus. They discuss how female remnants may be present as some men may be genetically mosaic – that is, they may have some female cells (46,XX) along with the normal male cells (46,XY). However, they point out that in this case, the 83-year-old man had only 46,XY cells (a normal male karyotype). The researchers go on to say that this man was thought to have prostate cancer but was later found to have adenocarcinoma. He had been placed on 25 mg. TACE which he took for ten years. It is extremely interesting to note that TACE, also known as chlorotrianisene, is a type of estrogen. It has since been discontinued from use.

A more recent study done in 2014 by Jabr and Venk addresses a case of abdominal pain in a 52-year-old man with a history of cirrhosis and hepatitis C. He had two previous surgeries for an inguinal hernia within a two-year period. He presented to the emergency room with excruciating pain in his right lower abdomen and pelvis. A mass was found attached to the urinary bladder, and it extended into the inguinal canal. The mass was removed and tested, and it was found to be positive for both estrogen and progesterone receptors. The findings were consistent with endometriosis. The researchers note that cirrhosis is known to be associated with high estradiol levels.

Jabr and Venk go on to discuss several other previous studies. Endometrial-like tissue was discovered in two men with prostate cancer, both of which had been treated with estrogen for several years. The researchers also point out that another man was diagnosed with endometriosis after inguinal hernia surgery. They hypothesize that inguinal surgery coupled with high estrogen levels may increase the risk of development of endometriosis in the male. They also state induction appears to be a likely pathway for the development of endometriosis. Induction is the formation of endometriotic-like tissue as the result of unknown factors, endogenous or exogenous, inducing change in undifferentiated mesenchymal or embryonic cells.

Most people think of endometriosis as a disorder that affects women only; however, it has been seen in men. It is important to note this as it may give us much-needed information as to what factors play a role in the development of this disorder. According to these few studies, it appears that estrogen (estradiol) may play an important role in the development of endometriosis and adenomyosis. I hope that more studies in men are forthcoming.

History of Adenomyosis and Endometriosis

The actual history of adenomyosis and endometriosis will help to clarify the difference between the two disorders. Scientists have been aware of the presence of endometrial-like tissue outside of the uterus for over 150 years. For decades, this tissue was referred to as an "adenomyoma", and its origin was not known. The first person to describe an "adenomyoma" in the literature was Carl von Rokitansky in 1860. Believing that the condition was cancerous, he called his finding "cystosarcoma adenoids uterinum".

In the late 1800s, von Recklinghausen was able to distinguish two separate disease entities which today would be called endometriosis and adenomyosis. He found some adenomyomas were inside the uterine muscle while others were found outside the uterus. He noted the adenomyomas inside the uterine muscle appeared to have glands from the uterine mucosa while those outside the uterus did not.

In the early 1900s, Thomas Stephen Cullen, an American gynecologist, published findings on what we would call adenomyosis today. His diagnostic criteria included "lengthened menstrual periods...may be replaced by a continuous hemorrhagic discharge...great deal of pain" (Benagiano et al., 2010, Diagnosis section, para. 3). He divided the disorder into three different categories since he believed endometrial tissue was present not only in growths in the uterine wall, but also in growths that occurred outside the uterus (known as endometriosis today):

- Adeomyomas where the uterus maintains a normal shape
- Subperitoneal adenomyomas
- Submucosal adenomyomas

During his research on uteri that were affected by adenomyosis, Cullen noted a "uniformly enlarged uterus about four times the natural size. On opening it, I found that the increase in size was due to a diffuse thickening of the anterior wall" (Benagiano et al., 2010, Historical Perspectives section, para. 7).

During these early years, adenomyosis and endometriosis were included under the same diagnostic umbrella. Another physician named Lockyer resisted the idea that adenomyomas located outside of the uterus contained endometrial tissue. He did, however, agree that abnormal growths occurred in many places including the digestive tract, gallbladder and kidneys. The subject of the source of the tissue was a point of contention for many years, but eventually Cullen's theory proved true.

In 1925, another physician named Frankl decided to name the invasion of endometrial tissue into the uterine muscle "adenomyosis uteri". He was also the first to clearly describe the difference between adenomyosis and adenomyomas. Frankl also worked with Sampson to show the similarities seen between adenomyosis and endometriosis. While examining the uterine tissue of a fifty-year-old woman who had adenomyosis, he noted similarities between his findings and Sampson's findings. He stated "This observation reminds one of menstruating uterine mucosa on the surface of the ovary, first described by Sampson. By the courtesy of Sampson, I had an opportunity of studying the original slides, and I confirm that both in his and in my case, misplaced uterine glands were seen filled with blood, undoubtedly menstrual blood" (Benagiano et al., 2010, Definition section, para. 5). Two years later, Sampson named the endometrial tissue found outside of the uterus as "endometriosis".

Recently, Kunz, Herbertz, Beil, Huppers and Leyendecker (2007) used magnetic resonance imaging to determine that an area of the uterine wall called the junctional zone (JZ) may be of utmost importance in the diagnosis of endometriosis. The group determined that the thickness of the JZ directly correlated to the presence of endometriosis in the peritoneal cavity. These findings point to the fact that JZ abnormalities may be involved in both adenomyosis and endometriosis. Interestingly, a thickening of the JZ has also been linked to infertility.

Today, several radiological findings may suggest the presence of adenomyosis. According to Benagiano et al. (2010, Definition section, para. 6), a diagnosis of adenomyosis "should be restricted to the presence of glandular and stromal extensions of more than 2.5 mm below the endo-myometrial junction on low-power field." Since that time, new studies have shown a thickness of greater than 12 mm of the JZ can be considered diagnostic for adenomyosis (normal thickness is 5-12 mm).

Bird came up with the current definition of adenomyosis (as cited in Benagiano et al., 2010, Definition section, para. 6):

"Adenomyosis may be defined as the benign invasion of endometrium into the myometrium producing a diffusely enlarged uterus which microscopically exhibits ectopic non-neoplastic, endometrial glands and stroma surrounded by the hypertrophic and hyperplastic myometrium."

Adenomyosis and Endometriosis: Myth vs. Fact

The following is a blog from Adenomyosis Fighters that summarizes the myths vs. facts regarding adenomyosis and endometriosis:

I have recently read some online articles about adenomyosis and endometriosis and have noticed quite a few misconceptions about these disorders. Since I recently wrote a book on adenomyosis after months of research into clinical studies, I feel it is necessary to write a myth vs. fact blog on these disorders.

Many misconceptions come from old information. Some of these inaccuracies are a result of a failure of medical professionals to update their current knowledge. I hope the following information will clarify the facts on these two disorders.

Myth: Adenomyosis and endometriosis are the same disorder.

False. Adenomyosis and endometriosis are similar, but they are not the same disorder. Both involved misplaced endometrial-like tissue (the tissue that is shed each month in the form of a menstrual period). In endometriosis, these endometrial implants are found outside the uterus on organs such as the bowel, bladder, and ovaries. Endometrial implants have even been found as far away as the brain. In adenomyosis, the misplaced endometrial tissue invades the uterine muscle and is confined to this area. It is important to note that many women suffer from both disorders at the same time.

Myth: Adenomyosis only affects women in their 40s – 50s.

False. This myth is rampant online. This used to be the accepted belief, but in recent years, this disorder is being recognized in much younger women. According to a 2013 study by Taran et al., "the clinical age at presentation of adenomyosis may be significantly earlier than previously thought and that early-stage adenomyosis might present a different clinical phenotype compared to late-stage disease."[1] The reason for this change is due to the discovery of the difference in width of the junctional zone within the uterine wall (will be discussed later).

Myth: Pregnancy will cure both adenomyosis and endometriosis.

False. Pregnancy will only subdue symptoms due to fluctuations in hormone levels. Once the pregnancy is

120

over, symptoms will return, sometimes worse than ever. Pregnancy is NOT an effective "treatment" for these disorders.

Myth: Adenomyosis/endometriosis is due to physical trauma earlier in the woman's life.

False. This is an antiquated belief that is completely false. Both disorders can now be seen clearly on imaging tests if the physician/radiologist is knowledgeable about the disorders. Bowel resections have been done on patients where the endometriosis has progressed through the bowel wall. Both adenomyosis and endometriosis can clearly be pathologically proven, so the idea that the disorders are linked to some kind of abuse has been proven to be false.

Myth: Adenomyosis can't be diagnosed until hysterectomy.

False. If you go to a physician who is well-versed in adenomyosis diagnosis and treatment, he/she should be able to obtain a diagnosis prior to hysterectomy. As mentioned earlier, it has been found that the width of the junctional zone can indicate the presence of adenomyosis. The width of the junctional zone, visualized on MRI, varies throughout a woman's cycle but in general, a normal width is 5-8 mm. Studies now show that a junctional zone width of 12 mm. or more indicates the presence of adenomyosis. In a 2011 study by Novellas et al., it was determined a thickness of the junctional zone of greater that 12 mm. indicates adenomyosis with an accuracy of 85 percent and a specificity of 96 percent. A study by Dueholm et al. states that the use of transvaginal sonography and MRI together gives the most accurate results in the diagnosis of adenomyosis.

Myth: Adenomyosis and endometriosis can be cured through hysterectomy.

This is only partly true – false for endometriosis and true for adenomyosis. Since adenomyosis involves only the uterus, removing the uterus will cure the condition. Since implants are found outside the uterus in endometriosis, removing the uterus will not cure endometriosis. Many adenomyosis sufferers become very confused when their symptoms do not resolve after having a hysterectomy, which is understandable. An important thing to remember is that in a lot of women, both adenomyosis and endometriosis are present. If your symptoms persist after having a hysterectomy for adenomyosis, you have probably been suffering from both adenomyosis and endometriosis.

Chapter 7 - Symptoms of Adenomyosis

"I fight for my health every day in ways that most people don't understand. I'm not lazy. I'm a warrior!"

– unknown

The following is a comprehensive list of all the possible symptoms of adenomyosis. Some women experience many of the symptoms while other women don't have any symptoms. In my case I had about seventy-five percent of the listed symptoms. It is also important to note that the pain associated with adenomyosis may increase over time and may become debilitating.

In my case, the most severe symptom was the pain associated with the abdominal cramping. I also had very long and heavy periods, most of the time twelve to fourteen days. Although it didn't happen to me, I have heard stories about how some women had to change their pad/tampon every hour due to the heavy bleeding and about how some women had to wear two pads at a time. I think most of us with this disorder have experienced that time when the bleeding was so heavy that the blood seeped onto our clothes.

I also suffered terribly with constipation during my period. I had a retroflexed uterus which means it tilts backward toward the rectum. Even though the position of the uterus isn't supposed to cause any issues, I sometimes wonder if the retroflexion played a role in my constipation. It seems to me that if my uterus was tilted backward onto the rectum and my uterus enlarged significantly during an attack of adenomyosis, wouldn't that place extra pressure on the bowel? The cramping pain and constipation were so bad in my case I thought I had a bowel obstruction. I still wonder that to this day. I also wonder if women who have an anteflexed uterus suffer from more bladder issues since the uterus is tilted forward toward the bladder. These are just my own thoughts. I haven't found any discussion about this issue in the scientific literature, but I would love to see a study on this aspect of the disorder.

Please keep in mind that not everyone will have all these symptoms, and not everyone will experience the symptoms to the same degree.

- **Menorrhagia** – abnormally heavy menstrual bleeding. Some people also call it "flooding". If you must change your pad or tampon every hour or so, this is abnormal. The amount of blood lost during a normal period is anywhere from 10-35 ml. One maxi pad can hold about 5 ml, so during a normal period, a woman will use anywhere from 2 to 7 pads during her whole period. If you are using many more maxi pads than this, it is abnormal, and you may be suffering from menorrhagia.
- **Dysmenorrhea** – severe abdominal cramping. It is normal to have some cramping during a menstrual period; however, the severity of cramping in adenomyosis can sometimes be as severe as the last stage of labor. This is not normal. Interestingly, according to Pamela Smith (2010), "studies have shown that women with dysmenorrhea produce eight to thirteen times more prostaglandin E2 than women who do not have painful cycles." Prostaglandin E2 is known to be one of the main causes of dysmenorrhea, and ibuprofen blocks prostaglandin activity which is why this medication is usually effective in reducing menstrual cramps.
- **Enlarged, bulky and heavy uterus** – the size of a normal uterus is 7 cm. long, 4 cm. wide and 4 cm. thick. The uterus can double or triple in size due to inflammation and the trapped blood inside the uterine muscle. The bloating associated with this uterine enlargement can make the patient look as if she is three to four months pregnant.
- **Tenderness or pain during a pelvic exam**

- **Nausea and/or vomiting** due to the severe pain associated with this disorder and/or hormonal imbalance.
- **A "bearing down sensation"**
- **Heaviness and pain in the legs** due to sciatica. The sciatic nerve runs from the base of the spine through the piriformis muscle (the large muscle in the butt) and into the thighs. From there, it breaks off into smaller nerves that travel all the way into the feet. Pain that originates in the pelvic region can be felt in the legs and even into the feet.
- **Pain in the lower back**
- **Bleeding between periods**
- **Spotting or a continuous bloody discharge** - This discharge may appear brown because it is old blood that has been trapped inside the uterine wall. This old brown blood may also have some mucus in it.
- **Painful intercourse**
- **Pressure on the bladder** that may lead to frequent urination.
- **Painful bowel movements during menstruation.** This may be due to pressure on the bowel from the inflamed and enlarged uterus. In addition, there may be episodes of alternating constipation and diarrhea. These symptoms are also indicative of irritable bowel syndrome, or IBS. Quite often, adenomyosis is misdiagnosed as IBS due to these symptoms, so it is imperative that you share ALL symptoms with your doctor, most importantly your gynecological symptoms, to improve your chances of obtaining a correct diagnosis.
- **Passing large blood clots during menstruation.** There have been reports of these clots being as large as the palm of your hand. Some women have described the clots as looking like a piece of liver. If you pass large clots that have this appearance, please report it to your doctor immediately. This is not normal.

- **Prolonged menstrual bleeding** – prolonged menstrual bleeding. A normal menstrual cycle should last about 4 to six days. Women with adenomyosis can have periods that last eight to fourteen days and sometimes longer. A good way to keep track of your length of your period is by using one of the many period tracker apps. One of these apps is called Period Tracker – Period Calendar Ovulation Tracker. It is rated with 4.8 stars, and it has over 70,000,000 users. In addition, it is listed as #1 in Health and Fitness in over 43 countries. If you don't like that one, there are many others that you can install on your phone. By tracking your period, you can give detailed information to your doctor about your excessive blood loss.
- **Chronic anemia due to excessive blood loss** - This anemia can cause extreme fatigue, heart palpitations and dizziness. If you have these symptoms, see your doctor. They will perform a blood test to see if you are anemic, and if you are, you may be prescribed iron supplements. These supplements should improve your symptoms.
- **Depression, anxiety and emotional instability possibly leading to suicidal ideation** - This subject will be discussed in much more detail in a later chapter.
- **Infertility, miscarriage, and possible myometrial ectopic pregnancy**
- **Migraine headaches** which happen most commonly during the week prior to menstruation.
- **Nausea, vomiting and diarrhea**
- **Extreme mood swings** due to hormonal fluctuations.

Additional symptoms

The following list are symptoms that women report on my Adenomyosis Fighters Support Page. These symptoms are not usually listed in medical sites such as WebMD™ or in scientific publications. I feel it is important to include these symptoms as they may be overlooked by physicians or be attributed to another medical issue.

- Feeling full after eating only a small amount of food
- Food aversions and/or food cravings near the time of menstruation
- Feeling of painful pressure in the pelvic region
- Weight gain even though the patient is exercising and eating right
- Inability to stand for long periods of time due to lower back and pelvic pain
- An acidic-type feeling inside the uterus
- Feeling that the bladder has not been fully emptied after urination
- Bloating after eating
- Interstitial cystitis
- Painful Pap smears
- Bleeding that can be continuous for months
- Increase in sinus issues/colds near the time of menstruation
- Butterfly-type rash or hyperpigmentation on face
- Excess intestinal gas

Chapter 8 - Complications of Adenomyosis and Endometriosis

"Courage does not always roar. Sometimes courage is the quiet voice at the end of the day saying, 'I will try again tomorrow."

– Mary Anne Radmacher

As I mentioned previously, fibroids and polyps also commonly occur with adenomyosis and endometriosis. In addition to those two disorders, there are other conditions associated with adenomyosis and endometriosis. In this chapter, I will delve more deeply into these conditions.

Infertility

Infertility has been reported in women with adenomyosis although no epidemiological studies have been done to confirm this finding. However, in animal experiments, baboons with adenomyosis have had infertility problems and endometriosis (Campo et al., 2012). According to Garavaglia et al. (2015), "The more and more frequent diagnosis in fertility clinics during the diagnostic work-up and its detection in baboons with lifelong infertility have suggested that [adenomyosis] may develop in young women and may have important consequences on fertility."

De Souza, Brosens, Schwieso, Paraschos and Winston (1995) report in women with painful and heavy periods who also had problems with infertility had a 54% incidence of junctional zone (JZ) hyperplasia. Seventy percent of these women never had children. Studies have also shown an increase in the risk of pre-term delivery in women with both adenomyosis and endometriosis. This could possibly be due to failure of deep implantation of the placenta due to JZ thickening.

Sadly, one study has shed some disappointing light on the success rate of in vitro fertilization (IVF) in women with adenomyosis. Vercellini et al. (2014) performed a meta-analysis of published data on this subject and found that "adenomyosis appears to impact negatively on IVF/ICSI outcome owing to reduced likelihood of clinical pregnancy and implantation and increased risk of early pregnancy loss" (Abstract).

The following are some of the factors that may indicate a link between adenomyosis and infertility:

- **Overexpression of HLA** - Ota et al. (1998) showed that women with adenomyosis have an overexpression of class II human leukocyte antigens (HLA). These antigens are involved in the production of cytokines and immunoglobulin, and these substances can act against phospholipid which may lead to either miscarriage or infertility.

- **Free radicals** – In adenomyosis, it has been shown that the uterus may contain an excessive amount of free radicals, and this may actually damage the fertilized egg. (Campo et al., 2012). According to Garavaglia et al. (2015), "the presence of high levels of intrauterine free radicals has a negative influence during sperm transport, implantation and pregnancy." According to Noda et al. (1991), there needs to be a low level of oxygen free radicals in the uterus for proper development of the embryo." This group goes on to say that free radicals in the uterus can cause the death of the developing embryo. Because of the presence of these toxic substances, macrophages or T-cells (types of white blood cells) will attack the free radicals which may cause an early miscarriage. One highly reactive free radical is nitric oxide. It is known to induce the COX-2 system which leads to high levels of both PGE2 and PG12. Ota et al. (1998) studied the levels of nitric oxide in the endometrium of women with adenomyosis and endometriosis and found that the level of nitric oxide was significantly higher in these women than in the control group. High levels of nitric oxide have been shown to reduce sperm motility and increase uterine peristalsis. Both of these factors could play a role in infertility. In another study by Jenkinson et al (1986), neural tube deformities increased in rats when high levels of oxygen free radicals were injected into the amniotic fluid.

- **Hyperestrogenism (estrogen dominance)** – When the uterus is in a constant state of tissue injury and repair (the TIAR system), this leads to higher than normal production of PGE2 which leads to the production of even more estrogen. This cycle also leads to the loss of action of progesterone receptors and even progesterone resistance. This state of hormonal imbalance has a negative impact on fertilization and maintenance of a pregnancy.

- **Hyperperistalsis** – the increase in uterine contractions seen in adenomyosis could possibly affect sperm transport and proper implantation of the embryo. In addition, the increased contractions may cause pre-term delivery and premature rupture of membranes. Since prostaglandins are overproduced in adenomyosis, and prostaglandins are involved in dilation and thinning of the cervix, this could explain why pregnancies may not be able to be maintained in some women with adenomyosis.

- **Altered immune responses** may be responsible for early miscarriages in adenomyosis. See "Autoimmune factors in Chapter 10 for more detailed information on this topic.

- **Abnormal junctional zone** – Campo et al. (2012) report in women who undergo in vitro fertilization (IVF), evaluation of the junctional zone thickness via MRI is the best way to predict implantation failure. This group also noted that if the patient had a JZ thickness of 10 mm. or more, treatment with a GnRH analog prior to IVF had an improvement in the success rate of IVF. GnRH decreases the expression of aromatase which is overexpressed in women with adenomyosis.

- **Dysregulation of proteins** – Liu, Duan and Wang (2013) used mass spectrometry and found twelve areas where proteins were dysregulated in adenomyosis. These abnormal protein expressions may cause the loss of normal rhythmic contractions in the JZ. This may play a role in proper sperm transport needed for a successful pregnancy. In addition, a study by Yen et al. (2006) showed some implantation markers that are seen during normal implantation of the embryo in the uterus are decreased in women with adenomyosis. They suggest this may be a factor in a decrease in implantation rate.

Frozen Pelvis

Frozen pelvis in the worst possible form of endometriosis. Also called "end stage endometriosis" or "terminal endometriosis", this disorder is caused by deep, infiltrating endometriosis, also known as DIE. Because of fibrotic tissue that is attached to pelvic ligaments, muscles and nerves, pelvic organs become frozen in place.

Endometrial-like implants that are present in the pelvic cavity respond to hormone fluctuations in the same way that normal, healthy endometrium in the uterus responds. As the implants bleed, the immune system treats the debris left behind as foreign invaders and attacks it. This leads to the development of adhesions. These adhesions can glue pelvic organs to the pelvic sidewall or to each other. They can also invade deeper into muscles and can affect the nerves. When this happens, tissues become hard like a rock.

In cases of frozen pelvis, patients may feel extreme pain during a pelvic exam. It can cause bowel obstruction and kidney swelling along with other disorders.

Symptoms of a frozen pelvis include:

- Severe leg pain
- Painful bowel movements
- Painful intercourse
- Frequent urination

Treatment involves multiple physicians from different specialties including a urologist, a colorectal surgeon, a vascular surgeon, and a gynecological surgeon who specializes in excision surgery. Surgery to correct this condition may last up to six hours.

Pelvic Floor Dysfunction

Pelvic floor dysfunction (PFD) refers to a disorder where a person has the inability to control pelvic muscles which leads to bowel problems. This disorder is common in women with interstitial cystitis.

During a normal bowel movement, muscles contract and relax rhythmically. In PFD, the muscles tend to contract more than they relax. This results in uncoordinated muscle movement which leads to problems with defecation.

Suspected causes of PFD include traumatic injury to the pelvic region or complications after childbirth.

Symptoms of PFD include:
1. Feeling like a bowel movement is incomplete

2. Constipation
3. Frequent and painful urination, involuntarily starting and stopping during urination
4. Pelvic pain
5. Painful intercourse
6. Unexplained lower back pain
7. Painful bowel movements

This disorder can be treated with physical therapy and medications.

Interstitial Cystitis

Interstitial cystitis (IC), also known as bladder pain syndrome (BPS) is a bladder disorder characterized by bladder pain, urinary urgency, and urinary pressure. To be diagnosed with IC, symptoms must be present for more than six weeks, and infection must be ruled out.

The symptoms of IC can be continuous or intermittent. Pain gets worse as the bladder fills with urine. In addition, pain can be felt in the lower abdomen, lower back, pelvic, vulva and vagina. This disorder may also cause painful intercourse.

Interstitial cystitis is two to three times more common in women than in men. Overall, about 3-8 million women are affected.

It is unknown exactly what causes IC, but several theories have been proposed:

1. A defect in the bladder tissue
2. The presence of inflammatory cells in the bladder called mast cells
3. The presence of something in the urine that damages the bladder
4. Change in the nerves that supply the bladder

5. Possible autoimmune factors

Treatments for this disorder include lifestyle changes (stress reduction and dietary changes), medications, injections and surgery.

Pelvic Congestion Syndrome

Pelvic congestion syndrome encompasses a disorder characterized by non-cyclic pain that lasts longer than 6 months that is due to varicose veins in the ovary and pelvis. Symptoms are usually worse when the patient sits.

When a patient presents with non-cyclical pelvic pain, the first tests will rule out some form of cancer. Once cancer is ruled out, this disorder may be considered. Once the diagnosis is made, there are treatments that have been reported to have a success rate of about 80 percent.

Pelvic congestion syndrome is treated by minimally invasive techniques using a transcatheter. Embolitic agents and/or coils are placed in the veins via the transcatheter to block the blood supply.

Ruptured Ovarian Cysts

Ovarian cysts are fluid-filled pockets on the surface of an ovary or in the ovary itself. There are several different types of cysts, and most are harmless. Most women have an ovarian cyst at some point in their lives.

These cysts are more likely to develop in women with hormonal imbalances or endometriosis. The type of cyst known to develop in women with endometriosis is called an endometrioma.

Most cysts degenerate on their own; however, some do rupture. Vigorous activity including sexual intercourse may cause a large cyst to rupture. This can cause internal bleeding and may cause symptoms such as severe pelvic pain, bloating, nausea and vomiting. In addition, large cysts may cause the ovary to twist and move which also leads to the above symptoms.

Ovarian Remnant Syndrome

Ovarian remnant syndrome is an unusual disorder that can occur after a woman with endometriosis has had a hysterectomy. Prior to hysterectomy in these women, the ovary is attached to the pelvic sidewall or bowel due to endometriosis adhesions. If extreme care is not taken to completely remove all ovarian tissue from the sidewall or bowel during hysterectomy, the remaining tissue will continue to react to FSH and will produce cysts and endometriosis. This will cause severe pain, usually on one side of the body. On ultrasound or MRI, the remnant will appear as an ovarian cyst.

Hormone levels will usually confirm the presence of an ovarian remnant after hysterectomy. Estrogen levels will be higher than normal in women who are not taking hormone replacement therapy. Also, the FSH level should be greater than 30, and if it is low, this indicates an ovarian remnant.

Bowel Endometriosis and Rectal Bleeding

Dr. Ken Sinervo of the Center for Endometriosis Care (2017) states that in his practice, as many as 60 percent of endometriosis patients have some kind of symptom related to the gastrointestinal tract. According to a questionnaire at his practice, "Intestinal cramping and painful bowel movements occur in approximately 25 percent of patients, constipation occurs in 35 percent of patients and diarrhea occurs in more than 60 percent of patients."

Dr. Sinervo (2017) states that only 10 to 15 percent of patients have endometriosis on the bowel. As previously stated, in many patients, endometriosis is misdiagnosed as irritable bowel syndrome. This happened in my case. I had a colonoscopy early on in my ordeal, and it was normal, so I was diagnosed with IBS. However, a normal colonoscopy does not automatically rule out endometriosis – it only means that the endometriosis has not penetrated the bowel wall.

Prostaglandins are one of the culprits in bowel symptoms in endometriosis. Prostaglandins cause smooth muscle to contract which not only plays a role in uterine contractions but also bowel symptoms. Cytokines and interleukins also contribute to bowel symptoms. Endometriosis can also cause rectal bleeding.
Another cause of bowel symptoms are adhesions. The bowel can become stuck to an ovary, the pelvic sidewall or the uterus by adhesions. Dr. Ken Sinervo (2017) also reports that bloating is commonly associated with adhesions.

As you can see, there are many conditions that can occur due to the presence of adenomyosis and endometriosis. Some patients may think that some of their symptoms are not due to adenomyosis/endometriosis when, in fact, they may all be traced back to these two disorders. Please remember that not all discomfort will be gynecological. Sometimes symptoms related to these disorders can be felt in the head in the form of migraines or all the way to the feet due to the involvement of the sciatic nerve.

Chapter 9 - Who is at Risk for Developing Adenomyosis?

"When the unthinkable happens, the lighthouse is hope. Once we choose hope, everything is possible."

– Christopher Reeve

Scientific studies and clinical observations have indicated that there are some risk factors for the development of adenomyosis. The role of these factors changes over time however. The first risk factor that I talk about below is age, and that has changed over the years as it was once thought that only older women were affected by adenomyosis. It is now known that the occurrence of adenomyosis in younger women is higher than previously thought. Keep this in mind as you read the following list. Studies and clinical observations may cause this list to change in the future. This list is accurate now only because of what we know today about adenomyosis.

- **Age** – Years ago, adenomyosis was thought to occur primarily in older women in their 40s or 50s. A possibility for the increase in this disorder at older age could be due to a woman's repeated exposure to estrogen. However, this line of thinking is beginning to change. Discoveries of abnormalities within the junctional zone through MRI have shown chronic pelvic pain and heavy menstrual bleeding in younger women may be due to adenomyosis. According to Taran et al. (2013), studies "suggest that the clinical age at presentation of adenomyosis may be significantly earlier than previously thought and that early-stage adenomyosis might present a different clinical phenotype compared to late-stage disease" (Risk factors section, para. 1).

- **Multiple pregnancies** – Women who had multiple pregnancies appear to have a higher rate of adenomyosis as opposed to those who have had no children (Taran et al., 2013). Also, Parazzini et al. (1997) report the greater number of births, the higher the risk of adenomyosis.

This could be due to the disruption between the endometrium and myometrium during pregnancy, or it could also be due to pregnancy hormone levels.

- **Prior surgery on the uterus** – Studies have repeatedly shown that prior uterine surgery may possibly play a role in the development of adenomyosis. The theory is that any kind of uterine trauma that could break the endometrial/myometrial barrier may lead to the infiltration of the endometrium into the myometrium. The procedures that may contribute to this problem include cesarean section (C-section), fibroid and/or polyp removal, abortions, miscarriages, spontaneous abortions and D&C. In fact, several studies have shown that D&Cs may be linked to higher rates of adenomyosis (Taran et al., 2013). In addition, another study showed a higher rate of adenomyosis in women who had cesarean section (Taran et al., 2013). Interestingly, Panganamamula et al. (2004) report that adenomyosis has been seen in a higher than normal rate in women who have undergone an endometrial ablation.

- **Antidepressant use** – The use of the antidepressant Prozac may increase prolactin levels and put a woman at an increased risk for adenomyosis. See "Hyperprolactinemia" in Chapter 10 for more details on the link between hyperprolactinemia and adenomyosis.

- **Treatment with tamoxifen** – In women treated with Tamoxifen for breast cancer, an increased incidence of adenomyosis has been noted (Taran et al, 2013).

- **Women with asthma** - A recent interesting study has linked asthma with endometriosis. A retrospective study using information from the Taiwan National Health Insurance Research database showed an "overall risk of endometriosis in the asthma group was 1.50-fold higher than that in the non-asthma group." (2018, Peng et al., Abstract). Prior to this study, the association between the two were inconsistent, but this study showed a clear association. Please keep in mind that this is one study, however. More studies need to be done to confirm these findings. I found this study intriguing in my situation because my maternal grandmother had severe asthma, and other members of my family have had asthma. I personally have never had asthma; nevertheless, the study was still interesting.

Although there appears to be some factors that may put women at risk for adenomyosis, clearly more research is needed. Interestingly, studies so far have shown that smoking, birth control pills and the intrauterine device have no association with the development of adenomyosis. However, the studies are very rare, so I take these results with a grain of salt. Since adenomyosis appears to be estrogen-dependent, I find it hard to believe that birth control pills have no effect on this disorder. In addition, I suspect that the finding that IUDs have no association with adenomyosis will change. There have been cases in which IUDs penetrate the uterine wall. Based on the previously discussed studies, this penetration of the uterine wall would disrupt the endometrial/myometrial border, so it would seem like this would increase the incidence of adenomyosis. I look forward to seeing what future studies will show. I strongly encourage more researchers to develop well-controlled studies to give us more information on the cause of this uterine disorder.

Chapter 10 - Why does Adenomyosis Develop? Results of Scientific Studies

"That's all. You don't have to do anything else. You just have to tell somebody else. You have to take whatever stigma people think that is there. You have to take it. It's not male or female. It has nothing to do with that. It has to do with, here's a disease you don't know about and you need to know about it. It's that simple.   It's   not   rocket   science."

[Whoopi Goldberg on endometriosis awareness from the 2009 Blossom Ball]

— *Whoopi Goldberg*

Many years ago, it was thought that endometriosis was caused by a "backward flow" in which menstrual blood would flow up through the fallopian tubes and into the pelvic cavity where it would implant on other pelvic structures such as the bowel and bladder. This theory has generally been debunked. As of today, the exact cause of both endometriosis and adenomyosis is unknown, but recent scientific studies have shed some light on this elusive question.

- **Hyperprolactinemia** – High levels of prolactin may play a role in adenomyosis as several animal studies have shown the disorder to occur in this state. Mori et al. (1991) first suggested that high levels of prolactin may cause adenomyosis, and Machida, Taga and Minaguchi (1997) report that infertile patients with endometriosis are always hyperprolactinemic. Sengupta et al. (2013) expanded on this idea by looking at the role of fluoxetine (Prozac) as a possible cause of adenomyosis since fluoxetine causes an increase in prolactin secretion. They were able to show a significant increase in prolactin levels in mice when treated with fluoxetine, and histological examination of the uteri showed evidence of adenomyosis. It is unknown if hyperprolactinemia is a factor in adenomyosis development in the human body, and further studies are needed to confirm the findings in this animal study.

- **Abnormal innervation of the endometrium** – Zhang, Lu, Huang, Xu, Zhou and Lin (2010) performed an interesting study in which they performed immunohistochemical studies on samples of the endometrium from women who had adenomyosis and fibroids. They were able to show that in women who had pain with these disorders, the nerve fibers in the endometrium stained positively for PGP9.5. They concluded that the results "suggest that PGP9.5 immunoactive nerve fibers appearing in the endometrium and myometrium of women with painful adenomyosis and uterine fibroids may play a role in pain generation in these two disorders" (Abstract).

- **Autoimmune factors** – Endometriosis is thought to have autoimmune factors that play into the development of the disorder. Because of this, Ota, Igarashi, Hatazawa, and Tanaka (1998) looked at autoimmune factors in adenomyosis. They found significant abnormal immune responses, and they specifically noted autoantibodies in the peripheral blood of women with adenomyosis. Wang et al. (2009) showed that interleukin-10 (IL-10) had a higher expression in the endometrium of women with adenomyosis. IL-10 is an anti-inflammatory cytokine, and this group suggested that the higher level of IL-10 may play a role in the lack of immune response toward the abnormal adenomyotic implants. There is also a high level of autoantibodies in the endometrium and peripheral blood of these women. In addition, there is overexpression of interleukins 6 and 8 (IL-6, IL-8) which contributes to higher estrogen levels leading to the lack of action of the progesterone receptors.

- **Hyperperistalsis** – Kunz et al. (2007) suggest hyperperistalsis, or abnormal uterine contractions, may

152

play a role in both adenomyosis and endometriosis. The researchers noted in women with endometriosis, hyperperistalsis occurred during the early and mid-follicular phases and mid-luteal phase of the menstrual cycle. In the late follicular stage, the contractions became arrhythmic and convulsive in women with endometriosis.

- **Beta Catenin** – In a study done at Michigan State University (Oh et al., 2013), the protein beta-catenin was found to play a possible role in the development of adenomyosis. Beta-catenin was first discovered in the early 1990s, and this substance was found to play an integral role in the formation of complex animal tissues Specifically, it is involved in cell adhesion formations in the maintenance and growth of the epithelium. It helps to regulate the growth and apoptosis (programmed cell death) of epithelial cells (Beta-catenin, 2015). In apoptosis, if a cell is damaged or not useful, the body automatically tells it to "self-destruct". This is a necessary function of the human body. If the apoptosis signal is turned off, cells would reproduce unchecked which can lead to a whole host of problems. Cancer is a perfect example of faulty apoptosis. Interestingly, certain mutations of genes that disrupt cell apoptosis of beta-catenin have been noted in many different cancers such as basal cell carcinoma, prostate cancer and medulloblastoma (Beta-catenin, 2015). More research in this area needs to be done to determine the exact mechanism of action of beta-catenin in the development of adenomyosis.

- **Vascular endothelial growth factor (VEGF)** – This substance has been found to have an increased expression in women with adenomyosis. Vascular endothelial growth factor is a potent factor in angiogenesis which refers to the formation of new blood vessels from pre-existing ones. This process is necessary when a wound is healing, but it can be problematic in other diseases such as cancer. The production of VEGF is known to be enhanced by estradiol. In addition, it is known to be expressed in endometriosis cells.

Hysteroscopy has shown that women with adenomyosis have vascularization that is irregular with vessels that are thick and dilated. According to Garavaglia et al. (2015), in women without adenomyosis, "the mean surface area, total surface area and total number of capillaries are all increased significantly in the secretory phase compared to the proliferative phase." However, this is not true for women with adenomyosis. According to Garavaglia et al., "the above parameters are increased in the adenomyosis group in both the proliferative phase AND the secretory phase..."

Estrogens are known to increase vascularization, and studies by Hyder et al. (2000) and Shweiki et al. (1993) have shown that the addition of estrogen to human cells induce VEGF expression. Another study by Cullinan-Bove et al. showed that when estrogen was given to ovariectomized rats, VEGF expression was expressed. According to Rocha, Reis, and Taylor (2013), "Endometriomas and red implants show the highest concentrations of VEGF" (Results section, para.3).

Another interesting finding is pro-angiogenic factors, including VEGF, are seen in increased levels in the peritoneal (abdominal) fluid of women who suffer from endometriosis (Rocha et al., 2013). Some anti-angiogenic drugs are currently being tested or possible use in adenomyosis patients in the future. Bevacizumab inhibits VEGF, and this drug showed some promising results in mice studies (Rocha et al., 2013). Other possible anti-angiogenic drugs include Sorafenib and

Romidepsin. Retinoic acid has been shown to have anti-angiogenic effects and appears to be useful in mouse studies. Progestogens have been shown to suppress the transcription of VEGF which may be one of the reasons progestogens have been useful in the treatment of both endometriosis and adenomyosis. The statin drugs have also been shown to have anti-angiogenic properties. Atorvastatin appears to inhibit COX 2 and VEGF in endometriosis cells, and Lovastatin® has been shown to inhibit angiogenesis (Rocha et al., 2013).

- **COX 2 and MMP 2** – In a study by Tokyol, Aktepe, Dilek, Sahin, and Arioz (2009), the expression of cyclo-oxygenase 2(COX 2) and matrix metalloproteinase 2 (MMP2) were investigated in women with adenomyosis. The group found the expression of both were higher during the follicular and secretory phases of the menstrual cycle of women with the disorder than in women without adenomyosis. COX 2 is an enzyme that is directly involved in inflammation. It is responsible for the production of prostaglandins which cause both inflammation and pain. This may be part of the reason NSAIDS are a possible, but not highly effective, treatment as NSAIDS block the production of prostaglandins. MMP2 is involved in the breakdown of the extracellular matrix. It also plays an important role in angiogenesis and promotes the mobilization of VEGF. This substance is known to be involved in the breakdown of the endometrium during menstruation. It is also interesting that increased levels of MMP2 are seen in melanoma, breast and ovarian cancers and that these increased levels indicate a poor prognosis for the patient.

- **HOX gene** – A study performed by Taylor et al (2000) looked at the expression of the HOX gene in the regulation of the development of the endometrium. They found that the gene expression was abnormal. This could indicate a problem with endometrial development at the molecular level.

- **Hypoestrogenism (estrogen dominance)** – see Chapter 10 for detailed information on this topic. Leyendecker et al. (2009) addressed the theory of excess estrogen as a factor in adenomyosis development through the TIAR system (tissue injury and repair). This group states that uterine microtrauma causes an increased production of estrogen in the uterus which leads to uterine hyperperistalsis. This constant microtrauma, operating through the TIAR system, may cause portions of the endometrium to invade the myometrium, leading to adenomyosis. Interestingly, a constant state of hypoestrogenism may lead to a loss of action of progesterone receptors and even progesterone resistance.

- **Exposure to Agent Orange** – Agent Orange was an herbicide used during the Vietnam War. It is a 50/50 mixture of two chemicals: 2,4-D and 2,4,5-T. The chemical 2,3,7,8-tetrachlorodibenzo-p-dioxin (TCDD) is a contaminant of Agent Orange that comes from 2,4,5-T. TCDD is of great concern in its possible role in the development of adenomyosis. According to a 2014 review of the literature on this subject by the Committee to Review the Health Effects of Vietnam Veterans of Exposure to Herbicides in Washington, D.C., TCDD may alter the ratio of progesterone receptors A and B, and it may block the ability of progesterone to suppress matrix metalloproteinase expression. The connection between TCDD and adenomyosis and/or endometriosis development was a secondary finding in a study that looked at exposure of this chemical in Rhesus monkeys. These monkeys were exposed to low levels of TCDD over a 4-year period, and they were found to have an increased risk of endometriosis. Even with these findings, the committee concluded that there was inadequate evidence to determine if there was a link between endometriosis and TCDD. However, that was reported in 2014. Since that time, more evidence has emerged that seems to link both adenomyosis and endometriosis to pesticides and herbicides (see Chapter 14). Future studies on this topic are warranted and would be extremely interesting.

- **Abnormal junctional zone** - Bergeron et al. (2006) suggests that the endometrium invaginates into the myometrium due to an abnormal or absent junctional zone. This group explains that weak smooth muscle fibers allows the endometrium to slip through into the myometrium. This invagination is supported by the presence of higher than normal estradiol receptor expression and Bcl-2 expression in adenomyotic tissue which in turn promotes the spreading of the adenomyosis further into the myometrium. According to Garavaglia et al. (2015), "[Bcl-2 and ER expression] may also promote other benign disorders: endometriosis, polyps, endometrial hyperplasia and uterine leiomyomas (fibroids) and this is probably the reason for which these conditions are frequently associated with adenomyosis."

- **Elevated levels of stress-induced phosphoprotein 1 (STIP 1)** – STIP 1 has been noted to be involved in the development of gynecological malignancies. It is a type of protein that controls the activity of heat-shock proteins which are active when cells are under stress. A study by Wang et al. that was published in 2018 showed that STIP 1 was found in higher amounts in women who had adenomyosis and/or endometriosis than in women without the disorders. The researchers also noted that surgical tissue from women with these disorders expressed both STIP 1 and matrix metalloproteinase-9 (MMP-9). Additional genetic testing showed that STIP 1 binds to a region in the DNA that controls the expression of MMP-9.

- **Elevated levels of CA125** – CA125 is a well-known marker for ovarian cancer. A study by Sheth and Ray (2014) has made the connection of elevated CA125 levels and severe, diffuse adenomyosis. They showed that in women with adenomyosis, the larger the size of the uterus in adenomyosis, the higher the level of CA125.

You might feel overwhelmed by what you read in this chapter. It just goes to show how complicated the human body is and how all these different proteins, enzymes, hormones, etc. all work together in the body and how a small imbalance in one area can affect all the other areas. Therefore we need even more studies. We need for scientists to develop many more studies based on these to come to a solid conclusion on the cause or causes of adenomyosis and endometriosis.

Chapter 11 - How is Adenomyosis Diagnosed?

"It is not OK to miss a part of your life because of pain and excessive bleeding. It is not OK to be bed-ridden for two-to-three days a month. It is not OK to have pain during sex. It is not OK to have major bloating or nausea."

(Address, 2011 Endometriosis Foundation of America Blossom Ball)"

— *Susan Sarandon*

In 2009, Benagiano et al. stated "...today a clinical diagnosis of adenomyosis is considered practically impossible" (Clinical Diagnosis section, para. 1). Although the disorder is still difficult to diagnose, thankfully some progress has been made since that article.

There is no consensus on what the criteria should be to diagnose a woman with adenomyosis. In hysterectomy specimens, most physicians agree that if there is endometrial intrusion of >2.5 mm. into the myometrium, a diagnosis of adenomyosis should be made. In women who have not undergone a hysterectomy, some irregularities have been noted in the junctional zone (JZ).

The Junctional Zone

Recently, the junctional zone has been of great interest in adenomyosis diagnosis. This area, also called the endometrial-myometrial interface, is the small layer between the endometrium and the myometrium (see diagram of uterus in Chapter 1). The JZ has been observed to contract in the non-pregnant uterus, and it is believed to be involved in the transport of sperm into the uterus to fertilize the egg (Novellas et al., 2011). In general, there have been consistent observations that a thicker than normal junctional zone points to adenomyosis. This thickening is usually seen in the posterior wall of the uterus and is an encouraging finding as this may help to diagnose the condition prior to hysterectomy.

The thickness of the JZ usually ranges from 5 to 8 mm. in normal, healthy, non-pregnant women. A JZ thickness of 12 mm. or more could be an indication of adenomyosis. Reinhold et al. (1996) showed a thickness of more than 12 mm. is a strong indicator of the presence of infiltration of the endometrium into the myometrium. Additionally, Novellas et al. (2011) state a thickness of greater than 12 mm. indicated adenomyosis with an accuracy of 85% and a specificity of 96%. This thickening can possibly be seen on ultrasound IF the technologist and the doctor are well-trained to detect this abnormality. According to Benagiano et al. (2010), MRI should be used to confirm the diagnosis. If the entire JZ is involved, the diagnosis is diffuse adenomyosis whereas if only a portion of the JZ is involved, the diagnosis is focal adenomyosis (Novellas et al., 2011).

The thickening of the JZ reaches its maximum width during menstruation due to the effects of hormones (Novellas et al., 2010). Benagiano et al. (2010, Adenomyosis section, para. 2) points out that "it is advisable to perform MRI for the diagnosis of adenomyosis after menstruation, as menstrual contraction waves can mimic abnormal JZ thickening."

However, there is a complicating factor here. As women age, the JZ normally becomes thicker. In fact, the junctional zone cannot be delineated in about 30% of post-menopausal women (Novellas et al., 2011). It should also be noted that the JZ is poorly identified via MRI during premenarche and during pregnancy. Benagiano et al. (2010) discussed in a review of adenomyosis that the term "junctional zone hyperplasia" should refer to JZ thickening without any other signs of adenomyosis. They point out this problem of JZ thickening as women age and concluded the term "junctional zone hyperplasia" should only apply to women less than 35 years of age. Gordts, Brosens, Fusi, Benagiano and Brosens (2008) clarifies this problem even further and even developed a classification system; however, it still needs to be validated. The classification system is outlined below:

- **Simple JZ hyperplasia** – a junctional zone thickness between 8 mm. and 12 mm. in women 35 years old or less.
- **Partial or diffuse adenomyosis** – a junctional zone thickness > or = 12 mm., high signal intensity myometrial cysts and involvement of the outer myometrium.
- **Adenomyoma** – myometrial mass, low signal intensity and an indistinct border.

A couple of other studies have looked further into the thickness of the JZ and the estrogen receptors of the JZ in adenomyosis. These studies are interesting and possibly very useful. I will mention them here as they may give researchers ideas for future studies.

A study by Dueholm et al. (2001) looked at the differences in thickness in the JZ of the entire uterus since the thickness can be different at different locations. They termed this the "junctional zone differential" and found that if the difference in thickness throughout the entire JZ was more than 5 mm., it indicated adenomyosis more effectively than an overall thickness of 12 mm. or greater.

Reinhold et al. (1996) looked at the thickness of the JZ in relation to the thickness of the myometrium. They found that a ratio of >40% was also indicative of adenomyosis.

Another interesting study looked at the estrogen receptor sites at the endometrial-myometrial interface (EMI, also known as JZ). Wang, Zhang and Duan (2010) determined the expression of estrogen receptor-α at the endometrial-myometrial interface in adenomyosis patients as compared to normal patients varied significantly at certain stages. They concluded, "the loss of periodic expression of ERα in myometrium of EMI of adenomyosis may be associated with an abnormal regulation of estrogen in adenomyosis" (Abstract).

In addition to the new abnormalities seen with the JZ, the following are tests that are commonly used to diagnose adenomyosis and/or rule out other disorders:

- **Endometrial biopsy** – This procedure is usually performed in cases of abnormal menstrual bleeding, no menstrual bleeding or bleeding after menopause. A sample of tissue is taken from the endometrium and sent to the lab where it is examined under a microscope for evidence of any abnormal cells.

  Before the procedure is performed, the patient is asked to empty her bladder. A sedative may be given. The patient lies on her back with her feet in stirrups. The physician inserts a speculum into the vagina and cleanses the cervix with an antiseptic solution. The cervix is then numbed either with a numbing solution or an injection. Forceps help to hold the cervix in place during the biopsy. Next, a uterine sound is placed through the cervix and into the uterus. This gives the physician information on the length of the uterus and where to take the biopsy. The sound is removed, and a catheter is threaded up into the uterus where several samples are taken. The samples are placed in a preservative and sent to the lab.

  After the procedure, the patient may experience some cramping and spotting for several days. NSAIDS can help with the cramping. Complications that may occur after an endometrial biopsy include infection, bleeding and a punctured uterine wall (rare).

  Although this procedure is useful during the beginning of a workup to determine the cause of abnormal menstrual bleeding, it may not be too useful in cases of adenomyosis. The biopsy only at a couple of places in the uterine wall. If the adenomyosis is not present where the biopsies are taken, adenomyosis may be missed. It's all about the luck of the draw with an endometrial biopsy and adenomyosis diagnosis.

- **Hysterosalpinography** – On the night before the procedure, the patient may be given a laxative, and on the day of the procedure, a sedative may be given. The patient is placed on her back with her feet in stirrups. A speculum is placed in the vagina, and a catheter is threaded through the cervix. The speculum is then removed, and a contrast medium is introduced into the uterus through the catheter. This medium enables the physician to clearly visualize the interior of the uterus. Some mild cramping may take place at this point. Pictures of the uterine wall are taken. When the physician is finished, the catheter is removed, and the patient is generally allowed to go home right after the procedure. The entire procedure lasts about thirty minutes. Although this test may be done to rule out other abnormalities in the uterus, it is not generally suggested for use in a diagnosis of adenomyosis due to its low sensitivity and specificity. However, Molinas and Campo (2006) suggest it could be useful since the endometrium may appear irregular with cystic lesions and abnormal vascularization. It appears that, at this time, this procedure would only be of use if the technician/doctor were heavily educated and experienced in the diagnosis of adenomyosis.

I personally underwent a hysterosalpinography during the years that I struggled with adenomyosis; however, the reason for the exam was due to the presence of a uterine polyp that had been seen on a previous ultrasound. I did not have any discomfort during the actual test even though I was warned about the possibility of cramping when the contrast dye was injected into the uterus. I did, however, experience severe cramping and bloating about thirty minutes after the test was completed. This occurred in the car on the way home in the middle of rush hour traffic. I did not expect this at all and was not warned that this might happen. Thankfully, my husband was driving at the time. I felt like I had to defecate, so my husband stopped at a fast food restaurant. I had a large bowel movement, and the pain decreased almost immediately (please note that I was not given a laxative the night before the test). I suspect the contrast medium irritated the uterine wall, and I had a delayed reaction to it. I don't want to scare anyone from having this test, but I feel it's very important for women to be prepared. If you have this test and suspect or know that you have adenomyosis, you may want to wait in the office for about thirty minutes or so to make sure you don't have a delayed reaction. It may also be advisable to have pain relief available just in case, and you may want to ask for a laxative the night before the test, especially if you have a history of painful bowel movements.

- **Hysteroscopy** – This procedure is used to look at the lining of the uterus and can be done using either local or general anesthesia. The patient is placed in stirrups. A small, thin scope is inserted into the vagina, moved through the cervix and then into the uterus. Gas or liquid is introduced into the uterus through the hysteroscope so the physician can better visualize the uterine lining. During the procedure, the doctor can take a biopsy, remove fibroids or remove uterine polyps if necessary. A hysteroscopy usually takes about thirty minutes, and it is usually done on an outpatient basis. Within the first twenty-four hours of recovery, the patient may experience some mild cramping and/or light bleeding.

This procedure is generally not useful in the diagnosis of adenomyosis since it does not look at the thickness of the uterine wall, but it may be a good place to start as it can rule out other causes of abnormal menstrual bleeding. Interestingly, Wortman and Daggett (2001) report that hysteroscopic endomyometrial resection may be useful in women who have undergone a failed endometrial ablation. However, it is important to note that 11.5% of the women in their study eventually required hysterectomy.

My experience with this procedure is about the same as a D&C. I was given a general anesthetic, and the procedure was done in a hospital. The first time I stood up, I felt dizzy and nauseous, but that passed very quickly. I had mild cramping and light bleeding as expected, but I was back at work after missing only two days. In general, I found it very easy to recover from a hysteroscopy.

- **2D/3D transvaginal ultrasound (TVS)** – This transvaginal ultrasound is performed with a full bladder. The patient lies on her back with her feet in stirrups. The transvaginal probe is covered with a condom and some lubricating gel. The probe is then placed inside the vagina. Images of the reproductive tract are seen on a computer screen. The technician moves the probe around a bit and takes images of the inside of the uterus, the fallopian tubes, and the ovaries. When finished, the transvaginal probe is removed, and the patient is allowed to urinate. Adenomyosis can be detected by TVS if the technician/doctor is knowledgeable regarding adenomyosis as this procedure is highly observer-dependent. In a review of adenomyosis by Benagiano et al. (2010, Transvaginal Sonography section, para.4), the authors state, "TVS should be favored as the primary diagnostic tool, although substantial experience and specific training is required to make sonography a useful diagnostic tool". According to Streuli et al. (2014, Section 1.1, para. 1), red flags include "globular uterus, asymmetry of uterine walls, poorly defined junctional zone, poorly defined focus of abnormal myometrial echotexture, distorted and heterogeneous myometrial echotexture, myometrial linear striations and myometrial cysts". In another article by Bromley et al. (2000, Discussion section, para. 11), the signs to look for on ultrasound include a "mottled heterogeneous appearing myometrium, a globular asymmetric uterus, small myometrial lucent areas, and an indistinct endometrial stripe". Although encouraging, these different studies use different criteria to diagnose adenomyosis; therefore, the data so far has not been too helpful. Although possible to diagnose this disorder by TVS, it will remain difficult to do so until one specific set of criteria is accepted. It needs to be noted that Exacoustos et al. (2011) report the presence of myometrial cysts on a 2D TVS can indicate adenomyosis with an accuracy of 78 percent and a specificity of 98%. In addition, this same group of researchers state adenomyosis can be detected on a 3D TVS with an accuracy of 85 percent if the junctional zone difference in thickness is >4mm. throughout the uterine wall. Although this sounds promising, Dr. Albee at the Center for Endometriosis Care states "Ultrasonography may identify sonolucent islands in the myometrium. But as with pelvic endometriosis, the ultrasound can't usually be specific enough to diagnose adenomyosis to the exclusion of other possibilities" (2016).

I have had many TVS exams during my battle with adenomyosis. Even so, this disorder was never picked up in my case. However, I struggled with this disorder from 1990 to 2007 when they didn't have the knowledge that they do today. This test is fairly easy and mostly pain-free. The worst part for me was having a full bladder. This can be especially hard when the office is running behind on appointments and you must wait. To deal with this problem, make sure the receptionist knows that you have a full bladder and that you can't wait too long. They should understand and work with you. Also, on a couple of occasions, the technician tried to get a good image of my ovaries, and she pushed the probe far to the side which caused some pain. If the test is uncomfortable, speak up. Don't be quiet – you are your own advocate in these situations.

- **Magnetic Resonance Imaging (MRI)** – This imaging technique has become extremely valuable for adenomyosis diagnosis. On T-2 weighted magnetic resonance images, the JZ can be visualized quite well. On MRI, there are three distinct zones that can be identified in the uterine wall. The endometrium has a high signal intensity. Underneath this layer is an area of low signal intensity which is the JZ. The myometrium has a medium signal intensity. When bleeding occurs in the adenomyotic tissue, the signal intensity may become high.

A normal JZ is about 5-8 mm wide, and the widening of this area to 12 mm or more is highly suggestive of adenomyosis. MRI has recently been found to be the most useful test for detecting adenomyosis when fibroids or other abnormalities are also present. According to Novellas et al. (2011), the presence of microcysts within the JZ or myometrium are indicative of adenomyosis. These cysts can vary from 2 to 7 mm. in diameter. However, according to this same group, these cysts can only be detected in about fifty percent of cases. An adenomyoma is easier to detect, but it must be differentiated from a uterine fibroid.

Dueholm et al. report the use of both TVS and MRI give the most accurate results in the diagnosis of adenomyosis. However, diagnosis through MRI is by far not an absolute. Dr. Albee at The Center for Endometriosis Care states "I am not hopeful that we will soon be able to rely on it to diagnose the isolated, scattered areas of glands lost among the muscle cells because of their small size" (2016). He also states, "MRI may be able to lead us to expect adenomyosis if myometrial thickness is increased or the consistency of the myometrium is changed" (2016).

Since I suffered from adenomyosis from 1990-2007, an MRI was never ordered in my case. Information about the thickening of the junctional zone was not available to physicians at that time. The new knowledge about the junctional zone should prompt more physicians to order an MRI if adenomyosis is suspected. In addition, insurance companies need to be aware of this and not reject coverage of an MRI in a woman with suspected adenomyosis.

Chapter 12 - How is Adenomyosis Treated?

"You are you because you love the way the world looks through your camera. You are you because of the way you love your friends and family. Not because some scar is on your body. That's a part of your history and what helps form what you believe in. not what defines you."

— A.M. Willard, Heated Sweets

This chapter will cover all the current treatments for adenomyosis. It is divided into three different kinds of treatments – surgical, pharmaceutical and alternative/natural. Depending on your case, treatments may involve one type or all three types of treatments.

Surgical treatments

- **Adenomyomectomy** – In this surgery, the physician will cut into the uterine wall and remove the adenomyotic lesions. It is also referred to as a wedge resection of the uterine wall and is performed under general anesthesia. This surgery has been linked to spontaneous uterine rupture during pregnancy, so a group led by Osada improved it by using a double-flap or triple-flap method when closing the uterine wall after the procedure (see Osada procedure in this chapter). Excision of adenomyosis will only be useful if the area of adenomyosis is focal and contained, but even in this scenario, the effectiveness is only reported at 50% (Taran et al., 2013). Fedele et al. (1993) report a high rate of spontaneous abortion after this procedure. In addition, there is a high rate of recurrence of adenomyosis. However, another study showed the use of this surgery plus treatment with GnRH analogs produced statistically significant symptom relief.

- **Colorectal resection** – Although women with adenomyosis only do not generally have to worry about this procedure, I add it here because in many cases adenomyosis and endometriosis occur together, and cases of deep, infiltrating endometriosis may lead to bowel resection.

  Two surgical approaches are used. The first one involves removing an entire section of the colon and the rectum. The other approach only removes a section of the colon but does not involve the rectum.

  Sadly, a French study by Roman et al. (2018) reviewed 60 cases of colorectal resection for treatment of deep, infiltrating endometriosis and found that these two types of resection ends up with the same rate of bowel disorders after surgery. Thirteen women in each group reported some kind of bowel problem two years after surgery in this study.

- **Dilation and curettage (D&C)** – This surgery is usually one of the first steps in treating heavy and/or abnormal menstrual bleeding. It is performed under general anesthesia usually on an outpatient basis. The surgeon first dilates the cervix and then uses a small spoon-shaped instrument to scrape or suction out the entire contents of the uterus. By doing this, he/she may also remove any polyps or fibroids that are found. If there is concern for cancer or endometrial hyperplasia, a piece of the endometrial tissue will be sent to a pathology lab for examination and analysis. After the procedure, there may be some cramping or spotting, but the patient is usually up and moving a few hours later.

  I have undergone a D&C many times due to heavy bleeding. The first time resulted in significant cramping; however, the nurse in the recovery room gave me plenty of pain medication. Also, I did have some bleeding, but this resolved within the first day. Overall, in my opinion, this surgery is easy to tolerate, and recovery is quick.

• **Endometrial ablation** – This surgical procedure destroys the endometrial layer of the uterus. It is not recommended for women who still want to have children. No incision is needed as tools for the procedure are inserted into the uterus through the vagina and cervix. An ablation is performed under general anesthesia. There are several different ways to perform this procedure. The possible methods used include microwave energy, high energy radiofrequency, electrosurgery, cryosurgery or heated liquids. Once the cervix is dilated, the method of choice is used to "burn" the endometrial lining. Patients can expect some mild cramping and a watery or bloody discharge for a few days after the surgery. It is possible to become pregnant after this procedure, but the pregnancy usually results in miscarriage. Therefore, it is imperative the patient use some form of birth control. An endometrial ablation may be beneficial to women who have superficial adenomyosis; however, those with deep adenomyosis may fail an ablation. In fact, according to Loffer (1995), 8 to 10 percent of women with adenomyosis will fail an endometrial ablation. In addition, Pageda, Bae, and Perkins (1995) reported that in hysterectomies of women who failed an ablation, 75 percent were found to have adenomyosis. Also, a large study on ablation failures was conducted at the Mayo Clinic in the United States. This study showed that women with adenomyosis had an increased failure risk and required either repeat ablation or hysterectomy (Taran et al., 2013).

If the woman has deep adenomyosis and has failed an ablation, hysterectomy is usually indicated. According to Benagiano et al. (2010), deep adenomyosis is considered if the adenomyotic tissue has penetrated 2.5 cm or more into the myometrium.

I underwent an endometrial ablation, and it failed. The procedure itself was fairly easy and similar to a D&C. However, I began to bleed heavily within 24 hours of having the surgery. After my hysterectomy, I found out that I had deep, diffuse adenomyosis, and this explained the reason for the failed ablation.

- **Percutaneous Microwave Ablation (PMWA)** – This procedure is like the endometrial ablation except that a needle delivers the microwave energy directly to the periphery of the adenomyotic lesion. A study by Yang et al. that was published in 2015 reported that after the procedure, the serum levels of CA125 and prolactin (PL) were significantly decreased for up to 12 months. In addition, uterine volume was decreased and there was no evidence of a decline in ovarian function. The authors claim that this kind of ablation has been used on adenomyosis patients and in women with fibroids "with satisfactory results." This surgery should not be performed if future pregnancy is desired.

- **Hysterectomy** – In the past, a hysterectomy was usually performed through an abdominal incision. Thankfully, due to surgical advancements, a hysterectomy is now done vaginally or using a laparoscope which dramatically reduces recovery time. The average time to perform a hysterectomy is two hours, and there are several different types of hysterectomy as detailed below:

  - **Total abdominal hysterectomy** – the uterus and cervix are removed. Fallopian tubes and ovaries may or may not be removed depending on the individual case.

176

- **Vaginal hysterectomy** – the uterine tissue is removed through the vagina.
- **Supracervical hysterectomy** – the uterus is removed, but the cervix remains.
- **Laparoscopic hysterectomy** – the uterus and cervix are removed through the vagina with the help of a laparoscope.
- **Laparoscopic supracervical hysterectomy** – the uterine tissue is removed through laparoscopic incisions.
- **Radical hysterectomy** – this type is more extensive than the total because it also removes the upper part of the vagina. It is usually done if cancer is present.
- **Oophorectomy** – removal of the ovaries. It is usually done if there is a history of cancer or if cancer is present.
- **Salpingo-oophorectomy** – removal of the ovaries and fallopian tubes. It is usually done if there is a history of cancer or if cancer is present.

This surgery has been the only way to diagnose and treat adenomyosis for more than a century. According to a study by Furuhashi, Miyabe, Katsumata, Oda and Imai (1998), women who have adenomyosis have a higher risk of bladder injury during a hysterectomy. Also, according to Benagiano et al. (2010, Hysterectomy section, para. 2), "most cases of failed vaginal hysterectomy for uterine adenomyosis are due to associated adhesions."

The following is a copy of a blog that I wrote on the Adenomyosis Fighters which explains in detail my experience with hysterectomy:

I recently started the Adenomyosis Fighters Support Group on Facebook, and I have noticed that a lot of women seem to have fears about having a hysterectomy. I want to alleviate some of those fears by sharing my own hysterectomy story.

I suffered from debilitating pain and very heavy menstrual bleeding for about seventeen years. During that time, I never received a definitive diagnosis. After a failed endometrial ablation, my OB/Gyn finally gave me the option of hysterectomy. I jumped on that option immediately because I was just so sick of dealing with all the pain and bleeding. I was terrified. I was terrified of the surgery itself, but I was also terrified of what would happen after the surgery. Would the pain actually be gone? After all, I still didn't know exactly what was wrong with me. Would I immediately go into menopause with those horrendous hot flashes, night sweats, and mood swings?

My doctor explained to me that she would only take my uterus. This would be done laparoscopically instead of vaginally. She explained that the laparoscope would go in at my belly button so they could view my abdominal cavity. There would be two tiny incisions on either side of my lower abdomen where she would insert two instruments that would remove small pieces of my uterus until most it was gone. She explained that with this kind of surgery, the very bottom of the uterus just above the cervix would probably remain, and this very small part may still bleed, so I might still have some very light periods after the surgery. She did not want to take my ovaries since that would send me into premature menopause. I agreed to this type of surgery.

Even though my doctor explained all of this to me, I was still scared to death. Again, I didn't have a diagnosis, so I wasn't sure if this surgery would take away the pain or not. By this point in my life, I had many surgeries, so I kind of knew what I was facing - signing in at the desk, filling out all the insurance paperwork, waiting until the nurse called me back, getting into a hospital gown, having the nurse start the IV....and then that long wait. Just sitting there, waiting, with my family members. This was always the hardest part for me. My heart raced, and my stomach was queasy. The only thing different for me was that the nurse came in and put tight stockings on my legs. I asked why, and she said, "to prevent any clots from forming in your legs". This just added to my stress...one more thing to worry about.

Finally, the time came to go to surgery. This was always a time of relief for me. When they gave me the drug to make me drowsy, all the stress just melted away. I was suddenly so drowsy that I didn't care what they did to me. Finally, my heart stopped racing, and my stomach settled. The stress was gone. Before I knew it, I was asleep. When I woke up, I don't remember feeling any pain at all. This was probably because I was so drugged up. I dozed on and off for a while. Next thing I knew, my family came in to see me. I don't remember much at first, but gradually, I woke up. I still don't remember much pain at all. A little while later, a nurse came in and removed

179

my catheter. I was nervous, but I really didn't feel much at all - it was quite easy. Later, the nurse asked me if I thought I could walk to the bathroom. I said yes, and I got up and slowly walked to the bathroom while the nurse walked next to me holding my IV bag. I was able to urinate on my own without a problem other than being a little bit dizzy. Several hours later, I was discharged and sent home. I slept most of that day. I still don't recall much pain at all. More than anything, I remember being a little weak and dizzy from the anesthesia, but I still had no problem walking if someone helped me.

The next morning, I got out of bed and walked into the kitchen where my mom was sitting at the table. She couldn't believe how good I looked and commented repeatedly about how well I came out of the surgery. I sat down at the breakfast table to eat, feeling pretty darn good. I was a little sore at the incision sites, but it really was minor. I ate breakfast, and a few minutes later, I had some abdominal cramping.

I need to stop here and give a little more background information on my ordeal with adenomyosis.

I had a retroverted uterus which means that it leans backward toward my bowel. One of the main symptoms that I had was excruciating pain with bowel movements during menstruation. The pain was so bad that at times, I had to crawl to the bathroom because I hurt so much. There were times I almost passed out from the pain, and at times I would end up vomiting. As my abdomen cramped, I would be unable to have a bowel movement. I could swear that at times, my bowel was obstructed from my adenomyotic uterus.

When I had this abdominal cramping after breakfast the day after my hysterectomy, I was disappointed. It was the same type of pain that I had before the surgery. I thought that the surgery didn't work, and anger, disappointment, and frustration just took over. The pain was fleeting, however. I went to the bathroom and had a bowel movement, and the pain dissipated rather quickly. Overall, it lasted maybe two minutes or so, and then I was back to my normal self.

That was the last time I had any abdominal pain! The last! I assume that this last bout of fleeting pain was a result of inflammation in that area because of surgery.

A few weeks later, I had a follow-up with my OB/Gyn. My mom was with me. She walked in to the room, sat down, and looked at me. "Well," she said, "I have some interesting news for you. The pathology report came back. You had a disorder called adenomyosis." She also told me that I may have also had fibroids. There was some question as to whether the problem was all adenomyosis or adenomyosis and fibroids. I have since learned that adenomyosis and fibroids are commonly confused by doctors. I was so happy to finally have a diagnosis that I sent roses to her thanking her for finally giving me an answer. Months went by with no pain, and I started to realize that this whole nightmare was over. Hysterectomy was the best thing I ever did!

For about five years after the hysterectomy, I continued to have extremely light periods as my doctor had warned me about. The periods lasted one to two days only, but there was no pain associated with them. About four years after hysterectomy, I began to miss periods. I knew I was in perimenopause, but I was told that I wouldn't be in complete menopause until I didn't have a period for a year. My periods were sporadic for several years. Finally, my periods stopped completely, and at age 51, I am in menopause. I did not take any hormones while going through the change. I had minimal discomfort during this time. I did have some sleepless nights, some night sweats, and some hot flashes, but all that was just annoying rather that disruptive to my life. Adenomyosis was hundreds of times more disruptive than menopause. I would take menopause any day over adenomyosis. Of course, that's just my experience. I clearly can't speak for all women!

So, I hope that this blog helps to alleviate fears in women who are facing a hysterectomy due to adenomyosis. Although each woman has their own experience, my gut tells me that if you can get through the pain of adenomyosis, you should be able to breeze through a hysterectomy. In my life, I have had ten surgeries - ruptured appendix, adenomyosis surgeries, three back surgeries, and a coiled brain aneurysm. By far, the worst pain I have ever felt is from adenomyosis. The only thing that has come even close to this pain is my ruptured appendix. The back surgeries and coiled brain aneurysm were a breeze to me. Women with adenomyosis truly are some of the strongest women walking the planet. If you can get

*through the pain of adenomyosis, you truly can
get through anything!*

- **Laparoscopy** – This surgery is done at the hospital, and
the patient is put to sleep via general anesthesia. It is
typically performed as an outpatient procedure.
Although not useful for adenomyosis, this surgery can
detect endometriosis, and since both adenomyosis and
endometriosis can occur together, this procedure may
be an option in treatment. However, it is now known that
excision (see Excision and Cauterization) is a better
option.

A small incision is made close to the belly button, and the
abdomen is filled with gas to better view the abdominal
organs. A lighted viewing instrument called a
laparoscope is placed into the small incision. If areas of
endometriosis are found, several smaller incisions are
made in the lower abdomen, and instruments are guided
in to burn off the endometriosis lesions.

Yeung et al. (2013) studied the effectiveness of excision
surgery as opposed to ablation (laparoscopic burning off
the endometriotic lesions). They state, "a high
percentage (84.6%) had received either previous
hormonal therapy or surgery by ablation as "treatment"
for presumed endometriosis, indicating that these
interventions are ineffective at suppressing or
preventing disease." Excision is clearly the better
alternative in dealing with endometriosis.

I had one laparoscopy done during my ordeal with
adenomyosis. The incisions are small (less than one inch).
Recovery took about one week, and I was given some
pain medication to take if needed. I don't remember
being in tremendous pain – just a little uncomfortable.
But that was just my experience. Another girl who had

the same procedure said she felt like she had just had a C-section. However, she described the worst pain in her shoulders. Pain in your shoulders after this procedure is due to the gas that they introduce into your abdomen to distend it in order see the uterus and ovaries during the procedure. After surgery, the gas rises as you sit up which leads to a sore feeling in your back and shoulders. To me, it felt like I had just been through a tough workout in the gym. The good news is that the gas works its way out of the body rather quickly, usually within a couple of days.

- **Magnetic resonance-guided focused ultrasound (MRgFUS)** – This non-invasive procedure looks promising as the recovery time is shorter and there is a lower risk of complications compared to other procedures. Using magnetic resonance imaging, a beam of energy is sent directly to the adenomyosis lesion which destroys it without injuring any tissue around it. This procedure also looks promising for those women who wish to preserve their fertility. Currently, magnetic resonance-guided focused ultrasound has been approved for use in the United States only for fibroids.

The fist adenomyosis patient to be treated with this procedure had no complications and conceived following the procedure. In addition, the procedure did not affect the pregnancy and delivery of the baby (Taran et al., 2013). According to a study done by Fukunishi et al. (2008), this procedure is effective at destroying most lesions of adenomyosis that are near the serosa of the endometrium. Also, symptom reduction as well as a lack of serious complications were reported. Kim et al. (2011) evaluated thirty-five women who had been treated for adenomyosis by MRgFUS, and they concluded the procedure was safe and produced a significant reduction of symptoms. However, in a study by Zhang, Li, Xie, He, He and Zhang (2013), high intensity focused ultrasound was shown to decrease symptoms in women with adenomyosis, but they noted that the bleeding and pain reduction was significantly higher in women with focal adenomyosis compared to women with diffuse adenomyosis. Currently, this procedure looks promising, but more studies are necessary to ensure its safety.

- **Myometrial reduction** – This procedure involves removing a large portion of the diseased myometrium by performing a wedge resection with uterine wall reconstruction. This surgery is not advised, however, because of the risk of uterine rupture in future pregnancy. In addition, the recurrence rate of adenomyosis is high (Osada et al., 2010). See "Adenomyomectomy" and "Osada procedure".

- **Osada procedure** – This is a modified version of myometrial reduction. After the wedge resection, the uterine wall is reconstructed using a triple-flap method. This method reduces the risk of uterine rupture in future pregnancies. In a study by Osada et al. (2010), 104 women who had severe adenomyosis were treated using this procedure. After the surgery, all 104 women had a reduction in heavy and painful menstruation. Over sixty percent of the women who wanted to become pregnant were able to carry their pregnancy to term.

- **Uterine artery embolization (UAE)** – During a uterine artery embolization, a small catheter is inserted into the femoral artery in the groin region. Tiny particles delivered through the catheter block the blood vessels that supply blood to the adenomyotic tissue in the uterus. A study of twenty women by Wang et al. (2010) revealed disappointing results. Only 15% of these women rated the procedure as satisfactory at six months, and 45% of these women were dissatisfied. Also, a recent review showed the recurrence rate of adenomyosis after UAE is high (Guo, 2012). A retrospective study by Siskin, Tublin, Stainken, Dowling and Dolen (2001) showed the satisfaction rate of UAE at a 12-month follow-up to be 92.3 percent. Postoperative MRI on these patients showed a significant reduction of the size of the junctional zone and the size of the uterus.

However, according to Bratby and Walker (2009), UAE is helpful in the short term, but symptoms tend to recur two years after treatment. Another study confirmed these findings. A 2005 French study by Pelage et al. followed 18 women who underwent UAE for adenomyosis. At 6 months post-op, 94% of the women reported improvement in menorrhagia. At 1 year, that number dropped to 73%, and at 2 years, the number dropped even further to 56%. Some of the participants elected to have hysterectomy because of failure of the procedure. They concluded that although the short-term results of UAE for adenomyosis look encouraging, the long-term results are disappointing.

- **Excision and cauterization** – Dr. Albee, founder of the Center for Endometriosis Care in Atlanta, Georgia has removed localized areas of adenomyosis with good symptom relief. Dr. Ken Sinervo also works at this same center and is an internationally recognized leader in endometriosis excision. The center performs LAPEX, also known as laparoscopic excision surgery, on endometriosis patients with incredibly good results. The procedure cuts out lesions of endometriosis without damaging surrounding structures. It is different than ablation or using a laser to "burn out" the lesions. Someone in the Adenomyosis Fighters support group explained it this way: Ablation is like mowing your lawn. You trim the grass (endometriosis lesion), but eventually it will grow back. But say instead of mowing the grass, you take a big truck and dig up the grass by its roots. The grass won't grow back. This is what happens with excision surgery. It's like cutting the endometriosis out – roots and all. Dr. David Redwine developed this procedure, and to date the surgery has been performed on over 5000 women from more than 50 countries. LAPEX requires extensive training and knowledge. According to The Center for Endometriosis Care (2017), "if the surgeon is not familiar with all the signs of endometriosis including those less common such as subtle areas of peritoneal tension, atypical clear vesicles, extrapelvic endometriosis, etc. then disease will be missed and left behind untreated..." The Center for Endometriosis Care (2017) also states that the success rates are high, saying "complete excision is possible in most cases and offers significant improvement in sexual functioning, quality of life and pain to many individuals, including in those with deeply infiltrating/fibrotic disease." However, excision is not necessarily a cure due to the complexity of the disease. The actual success rates of this procedure are 75 to 85 percent.

- **Presacral neurectomy** – Also called PSN, this is a procedure in which some of the nerves that supply the uterus are cut. The bladder may also lose some sensation after this procedure. The surgery is performed on the anterior side of the L5 and S1 vertebrae in the lower lumbar spine. Presacral neurectomy has the potential of damaging the iliac veins, the ureters and the sigmoid colon. However, this is rare. Dr. David Redwine states that he has performed over 220 presacral neurectomies without any reported injuries. A study by Biggerstaff and Foster showed that out of 27 women who had undergone presacral neurectomy, postoperatively 22 had no pain, 3 had a significant reduction in pain, and 2 had continuing severe pain. Dr. Ken Sinervo explains that about 85 percent of women who have had excision surgery improve. However, the other 15 percent who still have significant pain typically also have adenomyosis. Presacral neurectomy may help these women – in fact, about 75 percent of those who have had this surgery report less pain. This surgery has no impact on future fertility and pregnancy.

- **LUNA (Laparoscopic Uterosacral Nerve Ablation)** – Similar to PSN, during a laparoscopic uterosacral nerve ablation, the uterosacral ligaments are cut near the posterior cervix. This interrupts the pain signals that are causing pelvic pain; however, it only partially denervates the uterus. There is a possibility that a ureter could be damaged during this surgery, but there is low risk of damage to the bowel unless the cul-de-sac region is completely obliterated by endometriosis. According to Dr. Ken Sinervo, this procedure is rarely done anymore. He reports that symptom relief with this procedure rarely goes beyond six months or so. Presacral neurectomy is far more effective than LUNA.

Pharmaceutical treatments

According to a study by Streuli et al. (2014), non-steroidal anti-inflammatory drugs (NSAIDs), progestogens and gonadotropin-releasing hormone agonists (GnRHas) are the most commonly used medications to treat adenomyosis. However, according to Streuli et al. (2014, Abstract), "There are almost no well-conducted randomized controlled trials on the pharmacological treatment of adenomyosis, and the information collected from published studies is insufficient." The following pharmacological treatments are currently being used to treat adenomyosis:

- **Non-steroidal anti-inflammatory drugs (NSAIDS)** – These are possibly useful for women who still wish to have children. To be effective, they need to be started two to three days before the start of a period and taken regularly until the period stops. Keep in mind that some of these medicines may cause stomach bleeding if taken over a long period of time. Taking them with food and taking them for the minimum time possible may reduce this risk.

- **Aromatase inhibitors** – In both endometriosis and adenomyosis, there is increased activity of the enzyme aromatase. This enzyme increases the ability of androgens, such as testosterone, to convert to estrogen. In addition, according to Pamela Smith (2010), the expression of 17-beta-HSD type-2 is deficient in endometriosis. 17-beta-HSD type 2 is also an enzyme that converts the more powerful E2 into the weaker form of estrogen known as estrone (E1). It has been found that in endometriosis, there is progesterone resistance. Progesterone stimulates the production of 17-beta-HSD type 2. Because there is progesterone resistance and low progesterone production in endometriosis, 17-beta-HSD type 2 is not produced which leaves excess E2 present in a woman's body. Since endometriosis is estrogen-dependent, this explains why endometriosis develops in these women.

The following are all factors known to increase aromatase levels:

A. Elevated insulin
B. Elevated cortisol
C. Being overweight
D. Inflammation

Flaxseed, grape seed extract and red wine have all been shown to reduce aromatase levels.

In a study done by Soysal, Soysal, Ozer, Gul and Gezgin (2004), the use of aromatase inhibitors in addition to GnRH analogs in women with endometriosis showed promising results as it reduced the risk of recurrence for

24 months. Kimura et al. (2007) reinforced this finding and stated that this course of treatment may be useful in cases that were resistant to conventional treatments or in women who didn't want to have surgery. In addition, Badawy et al. (2012) showed that aromatase inhibitors are effective in reducing the size of adenomyomas and improving symptoms in affected women.

- **Progestins (progestogens)** – These hormones mimic the activity of progesterone; however, they are synthetic and come with side effects. Norethisterone, also known as norethindrone, is an example of a progestin. It is used for abnormal menstrual bleeding, PMS, endometriosis and some types of breast cancer. Side effects of norethisterone include breakthrough bleeding, bloating, breast tenderness, nausea, excessive hair growth, fatigue, depression and insomnia. This specific progestin interacts with many medications including but not limited to: rifampin, carbamazepine, St. John's Wort, tetracycline, theophylline, corticosteroids and thyroid medications. Its use is contraindicated in pregnancy.

Depo-Provera, also known as medroxyprogesterone acetate or Provera, is another progestin. Depo-Provera shots stop menstruation. This treatment usually controls bleeding and cramps, but it is not very effective in reducing tenderness.

Other names of progestins include Visanne and dienogest. Dienogest (DNG) has high selective progesterone activity and minimal androgen activity. A study done by Lee, Yi, Song, Seo, Lee, Cho and Kim (2017) looked at the safety of this progestin when used for more than 12 months in women with an ovarian endometrioma. The found "prolonged daily administration of 2 mg. DNG followed by surgery was associated with a lower recurrence rate of ovarian endometrioma and a reduced pain score and symptoms." Although promising, we must remember that natural progesterone is probably a superior choice to synthetic progestins (see Chapter 15 for more information).

- **Levonorgestrel-releasing intrauterine system (LNG IUS)** – Using this system (IUD) will cause the uterus to become unresponsive to estrogen as it releases a consistent dose of progesterone. Progestasert® was the first type of IUD of this kind in the United States. It was released in 1976. In 1990, Finland released the Mirena® which was approved for use in the United States in 2000. The most recent LNG IUS is Kyleena®. The first randomized trial for these IUDs showed that 90 percent of women reported a reduction in menstrual blood loss, and 30 percent of women reported a reduction in menstrual pain. Some women report spotting during the first 3 to 4 months after insertion of a levonorgestrel-releasing intrauterine system, but most women have stopped bleeding completely at 9 months post-insertion. Side effects include moodiness, oily skin, acne and weight gain. Once inserted, these IUDs last for about 5 years.

The process of insertion is fairly simple. The patient lies on her back with her feet in stirrups. Prior to the insertion of the IUD, the physician will do a manual exam to assess proper placement. First a speculum is used to open the vagina, and a tenaculum is inserted to hold the cervix in place. The physician then uses a sound to determine the length of the uterus. This will help in the placement of the IUD. The IUD is inserted and opens into a T-shape once in place. It only takes a couple of minutes to insert an IUD. Some women report pinching or cramping during the procedure, but this minor pain should dissipate rather quickly. A couple of strings hand down into the vagina after placement, and the patient is advised to check these strings often to ensure that the IUD is still in place.

In a study by Cho et al. (2008), this type of IUD was found to significantly reduce pain and bleeding, and the reduction of symptoms continued for 36 months. Sheng, Zhang, Zhang and Lu (2009) were able to obtain similar results in their study and also showed that CA125 levels dramatically lowered in these women. Mansukhani et al. (2013) report almost 50 percent of the women were asymptomatic after six months of treatment with a satisfaction rate of 80 percent (Abstract). Yet another study by Fong and Singh (1999) showed the successful treatment of a grossly enlarged uterus due to adenomyosis using this system. Fong and Singh also noted a marked decrease in uterine size at 12 months and reported the resolution of pain and bleeding in this woman.

Although the above studies sound promising, I must address the fact that I have read quite a bit of negative comments about IUDs on adenomyosis support sites. There have been quite a few women who have reported severe pain after the IUD had been inserted. Many women have stated they went back to their doctor within a week after insertion and demanded to have it removed due to severe pain. Other women have stated they were uncomfortable after it was inserted but pushed through the pain and eventually were pain free. Even though the studies look promising, many times what seems good in theory doesn't work out in real life. I strongly suggest you do your research before you decide to have an IUD inserted. Ask your doctor lots of questions, and even get a second opinion. Adenomyosis causes enough problems, and you certainly don't want to have MORE pain!

- **Continuous birth control therapy** – Low dose birth control pills (BCPs) with withdrawal bleeding of about four times per year may be helpful. However, no specific studies have been conducted in adenomyosis patients. In addition, since adenomyosis is an estrogen-dependent disorder, this avenue may not be optimal as BCPs contain estrogen.

  Having said that, continuous birth control therapy was one of the only treatments that actually worked for me. But remember, I had adenomyosis in the 1990s and 2000s before other treatments were available. It's really a decision on what works for you personally. Surgery may work for some, GnRH agonists may work for some, and continuous BCP therapy may work for others. The decision on which path to take is a personal one and should be between you, your family and your doctor.

- **Vaginal bromocriptine** – This substance has been used in cases of hyperprolactinemia. A study has recently been completed that investigated the effectiveness of vaginal bromocriptine in the treatment of adenomyosis. The results have not yet been published. See Adenomyosis and Endometriosis studies at the end of this book for more information.

- **Danazol** – This medication is an androgen. Its use has been effective in endometriosis treatment, but it is also known to have many side effects such as acne and excessive growth of body hair. Danazol increases the levels of androgens in a woman's body, stops menstruation, and starves the endometriosis-like implants of estrogen which causes the implants to degenerate. This results in a reduction in endometriosis symptoms. Other side effects include weight gain, a deepening of the voice, bloating, decreased sex drive, hot flashes and night sweats. Most women stop bleeding within two months of starting danazol, and the usual treatment is 3-6 months.

Thankfully, since the introduction of GnRH agonists, the use of danazol in the treatment of endometriosis has dropped dramatically.

- **Gonadotropin-releasing hormone (GnRH) agonists** – These medications reduce levels of testosterone and estrogen in the blood. Some common GnRH agonists include Lupron, Synarel, Zoladex, Prostap and Enantone. The usual length of treatment is 3 to 6 months, and most women will stop bleeding within the first two months. They can be given by injection or nasal spray. Side effects include mood swings, insomnia, depression, headaches, low sex drive, acne and bone thinning.

- **Tranexamic acid** – Also known as Lysteda, tranexamic acid is an antifibrinolytic agent. This means that it prevents blood clots from breaking down too quickly. Because of this action, it is effective as a treatment for heavy menstrual bleeding. This medicine should not be used if you have irregular menses, a history of blood clots, or if you are using any kind or hormonal birth control. In addition, this medicine should not be used if you ae taking anticoagulants such as warfarin or heparin or if you are taking medicines to help your blood to clot such as factor IX complex. Tranexamic acid is also contraindicated if you use tretinoin.

- **Mefenamic acid** – Also known as Ponstel, this medication is a pain reliever. Mefenamic acid may increase the risk of heart attack and stroke. Other side effects include an increased risk of bleeding, nausea, vomiting, constipation, diarrhea, headache and dizziness.

- **Endone** – a narcotic pain reliever. Also known as oxycodone hydrochloride.

- **Tramadol** – An opioid pain reliever also known as Ultram®.

- **ON-Q pump** – A non-narcotic pain relief system. This system delivers a local anesthetic to a surgical site through catheters. The ON-Q pump is used as a pain relief system after surgery. Narcotics affect the entire body which leads to side effects such as nausea and vomiting. The ON-Q pump is a better alternative because it delivers the anesthetic directly to the surgical site, and the medication does not affect the whole body. This leads to a shorter recovery time, less grogginess and fewer side effects.

- **Gabapentin** – Also known as Neurontin, Gralise, Horizant and Gabarone, this medication is an anti-epileptic drug. It is used to treat seizures, nerve pain and hot flashes. Restless leg syndrome can be treated with the Horizant brand only. This medication is a cheaper alternative to Lyrica. Side effects include suicidal thoughts, moodiness, headaches, vision problems, dizziness and sleepiness. Suddenly stopping gabapentin can cause severe withdrawal symptoms.

- **Muscle relaxers** – Garavaglia et al. (2010) state that a muscle relaxer may help uterine hyperperistalsis.

Alternative/Natural Treatments

- **Natural bio-identical and bio-available progesterone cream** – Dr. John Lee coined the term "estrogen dominance". He suggests the use of bio-identical progesterone cream in cases of estrogen dominance, starting on day 8 and ending on day 26 of the menstrual cycle. Dr. John Lee's site (ww.johnleemd.com, 2016) has loads of information about hormonal imbalance, and it is well worth the time to check it out. He states synthetic progesterone (progestogens, progestins) is not the way to go in trying to balance hormone levels He explains that synthetic hormones act differently in the body as compared to bio-identical hormones and explains how xenoestrogens (dangerous man-made chemicals that act like estrogen in the body) upset hormone balance. He also explains that if the progesterone isn't bio-identical, it can't effectively bind to the progesterone receptors. When taken by mouth, synthetic progestins bind to protein in the liver which makes them water soluble. This is a problem since hormones are lipophilic meaning they work in fat, not water. Once they become water soluble, they cannot bind to the progesterone receptors and are readily excreted through the urine. Bio-identical progesterone cream is different in that it is absorbed directly into the skin and into fat where it can work effectively. Dr. Lee states that improvement may be seen in two months, but it may also take up to six months. For a more detailed discussion of progesterone cream, see Chapter 15.

- **CBD oil** – Also known as cannabidiol, this substance is found in the marijuana (cannabis) plant. Marijuana contains both THC, which gives the user the "high" and CBD, which does not give the user the "high". Most CBD is found in hemp which is the least processed form of the plant.

According to Jon Johnson of Medical News Today, "A study published in the Journal of Experimental Medicine found that CBD significantly reduced chronic inflammation and pain in some mice and rats."

CBD is not legal in all areas of the United States, and most cases require a prescription for use. CBD is mostly well-tolerated but may cause tiredness and diarrhea.

- **Crystal Star Women's Best Friend Herbal Supplement** – The first time I heard about this supplement was on my adenomyosis support website as one of the ladies had tremendous relief using it. I researched it and was quite impressed.

   This supplement contains wonderful herbs that may help adenomyosis patients (see Chapter 20) such as goldenseal, wild yam, cramp bark, dandelion, black cohosh, dong quai, red raspberry and blessed thistle.

   According to the product's webpage on Amazon (2018), this supplement "helps strengthen, cleanse and normalize the ovarian-uterine area. Takes down discomfort and swelling so you start feeling better...helping to reduce excess estrogen...stimulates liver activity for improved estrogen metabolism. Supports your body's natural detoxification processes to clear congested wastes while reducing symptoms like abnormal bleeding."

- **Castor oil packs** – Castor oil is derived from the castor bean plant (Ricinus communic). It has been used since the times of the Ancient Egyptians. Castor oil is known to boost the immune system by increasing the number of white blood cells. Ninety percent of the fatty acids in castor oil is ricinoleic acid which is known to fight skin disorders, support the lymphatic system, increase circulation, help balance hormones and induce labor. This product is used in many skin products because of its skin-conditioning properties. Due to its ability to induce labor, pregnant women should avoid the use of castor oil.

- **Pelvic floor therapy** – physical therapists do this type of therapy. They use the following techniques to relax and strengthen pelvic floor muscles:

  Myofascial release
  Pelvic floor muscle EMG/TENS
  Stretching and relaxation exercises
  Biofeedback
  Deep tissue massage
  Craniosacral therapy

- **Yoga for Endometriosis** – A lady by the name of Allannah developed this type of yoga specifically for those suffering from endometriosis. Allannah was diagnosed with stage 4 endometriosis and adenomyosis after which she spent 5 years in formal training in yoga instruction and therapy. Her classes can be found online at www.yogayin.com/endometriosis-yoga/. Her premium classes are $10, but there are also some free videos available.

- **Heating pad**

- **Exercise** – Even though adenomyosis sufferers feel awful for about two weeks every month, exercise can be incredibly beneficial on those days when you feel decent enough to do so. Did you know exercise increases life expectancy? For every two hours you work out, it adds about one hour on to your life! Obesity has been linked to an increased production of aromatase which lead to an increased production of estrogen. This is one of the most important reasons for adenomyosis sufferers to try to exercise at least three times a week for thirty minutes.

Do you have problems trying to exercise three times a week? You don't have to go to a gym. Just make the effort to be a little more active during the day. Here are some helpful tips:

- Buy a FitBit®. This has helped me tremendously as it keeps me motivated. The goal for the number of steps per day is 10,000. That sounds like a lot, but it's not too hard to reach that goal. Checking on the number of steps you've taken during the day will keep you motivated to move more, and you can become friends online with other FitBit® users who can keep you motivated as well.
- Workout or walk with a friend. Exercising with someone else will keep you accountable.
- When shopping, park farther away from the store than you usually do. A little extra walking will earn you more steps on your FitBit®.
- Take the stairs instead of the elevator. This will also add more steps on your FitBit®.
- Try to get your workout/walking done in the morning or early afternoon. Exercising right before bedtime may interrupt your ability to get a good night of sleep.
- Do sit-ups, leg raises or just stretch while watching television.
- Gardening, shoveling snow or raking leaves are all good forms of exercise.

Exercise also has other benefits that may help adenomyosis sufferers. One great benefit is that it raises serotonin levels and will give you a sense of well-being. Since increased serotonin levels improves mood, it may help those who suffer from depression and mood swings. It also improves mental health and promotes more restful sleep.

It is important to lift light weights in addition to getting aerobic exercise. As a woman ages and especially near menopause, bone health becomes a concern. One way to prevent osteoporosis is by lifting light weights as part of your exercise regime. Lifting weights, even light ones, slows the loss of bone density. Additionally, increasing muscle mass helps with weight loss. The more muscle you have, the more calories you burn at rest. That's just one more great reason to lift weights!

Finally, there are other benefits of exercise that are just good for overall health. Exercise boosts HDL (good cholesterol) and reduces LDL (bad cholesterol). This will help keep your heart and cardiovascular system healthy. Exercise also reduces the risk of type 2 diabetes and some forms of cancer. Exercise also alleviates depression. So, when you are feeling strong enough, try to exercise. If you can get at east thirty minutes of exercise three times per week, you should feel better, and your body may become better equipped to deal with adenomyosis.

- **Stress reduction** – see Chapter 21.

- **Antioxidant therapy** – Garavaglia et al. (2010) states "in order to reduce the free radicals, patients could receive an antioxidant therapy such as vitamin E."

- **Acupuncture** – Acupuncture is a Chinese technique based on the belief that the life energy force, or chi, flows along twelve major pathways called meridians. Acupuncture points are located along these meridians. When tiny needles are inserted into the acupuncture points, or acupoints, chi flow is restored resulting in reduced pain and overall better health. Several scientific studies have shown that meridians and acupoints do exist. This technique has been shown to reduce pain through the release of endorphins and enkephalins, the body's natural painkillers. No more than ten to twelve needles are placed during a visit, and the needles are left in place for about 20-30 minutes. Overall, the procedure is painless.

- **Craniosacral therapy** – This type of therapy involves the manipulation of the skull in order to improve the flow of cerebrospinal fluid (CSF) around the brain and spinal cord. Therapists monitor the pressure changes of the CSF and any abnormal stress or pressure is released through manipulation techniques. According to Burton Goldberg, "Individuals who experience craniosacral treatment describe profound states of relaxation, of feeling lighter and more integrated." Craniosacral therapy is used to treat chronic pain, disabling headaches, swelling and many other disorders.

Section III

Chapter 13 - What is Estrogen Dominance?

"The current level of chemicals in the food and water supply and the indoor and outdoor environment has lowered our threshold of resistance to disease and has altered our body's metabolism, causing enzyme dysfunction, nutritional deficiencies, and hormonal imbalances."

-Dr. Marshall Mandell

Estrogen dominance is a condition where the progesterone to estrogen ratio is too low. In other words, there is not enough progesterone present to counter the effects of estrogen. This can lead to a whole host of health issues, most notably breast cancer. Pamela Smith (2010) states in her book, *What You Must Know About Women's Hormones,* "if you have PMS, postpartum depression, fibroids or fibrocystic breast disease, there is a good chance that your progesterone-to-estrogen ratio is too low." Today, this abnormal ratio is seen in both endometriosis and adenomyosis. The condition is usually observed and treated by natural health practitioners and not recognized my mainstream medicine. Most of the time, progesterone levels are not tested during regular hormonal testing by a family practitioner or OB/Gyn. This needs to change as progesterone plays such an important role in hormone balance.

Estrogen and progesterone expression defects have been found in women with adenomyosis. A study by Campo, Campo and Benagiano (2012) showed that the overexpression of interleukin-6 (IL-6) in adenomyosis could lead to increased estrogen receptor expression. The group explained that estrogen and progesterone expression in women with adenomyosis are different than in women with normal uteri. In addition, they note because there is overexpression of cytochrome P450 in women with adenomyosis, this can contribute to overexpression of local estrogen production. Also, a defect in progesterone receptor sites was observed. This could explain why so many women with adenomyosis also suffer from estrogen dominance.

Another interesting study regarding estrogen expression in adenomyotic tissue was performed in 2014 by Yamanaka et al. The group notes aromatase and estrogen sulphatase levels are higher in adenomyotic tissue. Aromatase is an enzyme that is involved in the conversion of androgens to estrogen. Scientists are looking into ways to block aromatase as a way of inhibiting the production of estrogen. Yamanaka et al. (2014) states this high level of aromatase suggests a higher sensitivity to estrogen in adenomyotic tissue. Also, they note adenomyotic cells appear to be resistant to apoptosis (programmed cell death). The group goes on to say some progestins appear to improve symptoms, so they decided to look at the effects of two progesterone agents on adenomyotic tissue. One exciting finding was both endogenous progesterone and dienogest (a synthetic progestin) increased apoptosis of adenomyotic cells. They concluded both endogenous progesterone and dienogest "directly inhibit cellular proliferation and also induce apoptosis in human adenomyotic stromal cells" (Comment section, para. 4). The researchers suggest dienogest may be useful in the treatment of adenomyosis.

The abnormal ratio between progesterone and estrogen is typically not picked up by routine laboratory testing as the ratio between these two hormones is not calculated, especially if progesterone is not included in the testing. In estrogen dominance, both estrogen and progesterone levels can be in the "normal" range, but the ratio of progesterone to estrogen can be out of range. The following is a measurement of my levels several years ago when I was struggling with gynecological issues. The test was performed at ZRT laboratories:

Estradiol	2.3	In range (normal is 1.3-3.3)
Progesterone	154	In range (normal is 75-270)
Ratio Pg/E2	67	**Out of range (normal is 100-500)**

Note: Pg stands for progesterone, E2 stands for estradiol

As you can see, this condition can be easily missed if the ratio of progesterone to estrogen is not calculated. Hormonal balance has largely been underestimated in the past as a cause of gynecological disorders. Today the prevalence of estrogen dominance in the U.S. has been reported to be close to fifty percent. It has been reported that from age 35 to age 50, the level of estrogen in a woman's body will decline by about thirty-five percent while during that same period, the progesterone level will decline by seventy-five percent (Biomedic Labs Rx, What is Estrogen Dominance section, para. 3). So, as you can see, estrogen dominance is of utmost concern as a woman ages.

The following is a list of some of the possible causes of estrogen dominance:

- **Adrenal fatigue** – see Chapters 3 and 21.
- **Anovulation** – When a woman does not ovulate, the corpus luteum will not develop. If the corpus luteum in not present, no progesterone will be produced in the second half of the cycle which leads to an estrogen dominant condition.
- **Exposure to xenoestrogens** – see Chapter 14.
- **Hysterectomy**
- **Impaired immune system**
- **Lack of exercise**
- **Luteal insufficiency** – This condition occurs when the corpus luteum does not produce enough progesterone to offset estrogen that is present in a woman's body during the luteal phase of the menstrual cycle. Clearly, this will lead to an estrogen dominant condition. In a study by Prior et al. (1992), out of 18 women with an average age of 29, seven were not ovulating and were not producing progesterone. This condition has been associated with the use of birth control pills.
- **Medications**
- **Premenopause and menopause**

- Obesity
- Ovarian tumors
- **Polycystic ovarian syndrome** – This condition occurs when a woman has an excessively high level of androgens in her body. When a woman does not ovulate, cysts form on the ovaries. These cysts produce androgens. Although the cause is not known, there has been a link to insulin. Many women with PCOS also have insulin resistance. Symptoms include missed or light periods, infertility, acne, excessive body hair and weight gain. The disorder can be diagnosed through blood tests that measure hormone levels and by ultrasound. Treatments include medications for diabetes, medications to induce ovulation, birth control pills, a healthy diet and exercise.
- **Poor diet** - lack of omega-3 fatty acids, excessive refined carbohydrates, low fiber
- **Stress**
- **Thyroid disorders**

The following is a list of some of the possible symptoms of estrogen dominance:

- Adenomyosis
- Allergies
- Anxiety
- Asthma
- Autoimmune disorders such as Lupus, Sjögren's disease and thyroiditis
- Bloating
- Blood clots
- Breast cancer
- Cold hands and feet
- Cravings for carbohydrates
- Decreased sex drive
- Depression

- Digestive problems
- Dry eyes
- Endometrial cancer
- Endometrial polyps
- Endometriosis
- Fatigue
- Fibrocystic breast disease
- Foggy thinking
- Gallbladder issues
- Hair loss
- Headaches, including premenstrual migraines – Estrogen dominance experts Lee in Hopkins (2004) state "When migraine headaches occur with regularity in women at premenstrual times, they are most likely due to estrogen dominance". They report that hundreds of women have been helped or cured with the use of natural progesterone cream.
- Heavy menstrual bleeding
- Hypoglycemia
- Infertility
- Irregular menstrual cycles
- Irritability
- Insomnia
- Memory loss
- Mineral deficiencies, especially magnesium and zinc
- Miscarriage
- Mood swings
- Osteoporosis
- Ovarian cysts
- Painful menstrual periods
- Premenopausal bone loss
- Premenstrual syndrome
- Prolonged menstrual bleeding
- Polycystic ovarian syndrome
- Sinus congestion
- Slow metabolism

- Spotting between periods
- Stroke
- Thyroid issues
- Unwanted hair growth
- Uterine cancer
- Uterine fibroids
- Weight gain in the abdomen, hips and thighs

Chapter 14 - Xenoestrogens

"Over four hundred pesticides are currently licensed for use on America's foods, and every year over 2.5 billion pounds are dumped on crop lands, forests, lawns, and fields."

-Burton Goldberg

Xenoestrogens are man-made chemicals that have estrogen-like activity in the human body. They are considered dangerous because they can cause endocrine disruption (altering the function of hormones) which can lead to a whole host of reproductive health problems. Some scientists and doctors believe that xenoestrogens are harmless to humans and animals because we are routinely exposed to low levels of these chemicals without any adverse effects. However, it has been shown that the effects of xenoestrogens are additive, and if we are continually exposed to low levels of many different xenoestrogens, it could possible lead to problems. According to a study by Bulayeva and Watson (2004), low levels of these chemicals may be more toxic than previously thought. The authors state, "these very low effective doses for xenoestrogens demonstrate that many environmental contamination levels previously thought to be subtoxic may very well exert significant signal- and endocrine-disruptive effects, discernable only when the appropriate mechanism is assayed" (Discussion section, para. 3).

Some of the most dangerous xenoestrogens are herbicides and pesticides. Elizabeth Lipski states in her book, Digestive Wellness (2000), "The average person consumes one pound of these chemicals each year. These pesticides have neurotoxic effects and can cause damage to our nervous systems."

An interesting study was done in Maine called "The Body Burden Study." According to Marcelle Pick in her book, *Is it Me or My Hormones*, the researchers "decided to conduct a study ...in which they had themselves tested for heavy metals. To their astonishment, they discovered that every single one of them had abnormally high levels of these toxic compounds. Even the 26-year-old woman who had initiated the study, young as she was, had accumulated quite a body burden already."

The following is a list of some of the most dangerous and recognized xenoestrogens. Many of these chemicals have been banned but many are still being used today. Also, some of the banned chemicals are still present in the environment since they do not break down easily. Women who suffer from adenomyosis are advised to educate themselves on these chemicals and, although impossible to avoid completely, try to do their best to decrease exposure.

1. **4-methylbenzylidine camphor (4-MBC)** – This substance is used in sunscreen. In addition to being an endocrine disruptor, it may also play a role in hypothyroidism. Margaret Schlumpf headed a study in Zurich, Switzerland at the Institute of Pharmacology and Toxicology in 2008. She and her colleagues found that 4-MBC applied to rat skin doubled the rate of growth in uterine tissue before puberty. Its use is approved in Europe and Canada, but it is banned in the United States and Japan.

2. **Alkyl phenols (nonylphenols)** – These substances have been shown to have clear estrogen activity. They are found in adhesives, carbonless copy paper, detergents, fire retardant materials, fragrances, fuels, lubricants, oil field chemicals and tires. The use of alkyl phenols in Europe is restricted.

3. **Atrazine** – Atrazine is an herbicide that is used on corn, sugarcane and other crops to control weed growth. It has also been used on golf courses and lawns. In 2014, atrazine was the second most widely used herbicide in the United States, and it is the most commonly detected herbicide in drinking water. Studies have shown it to be

an endocrine disruptor; however, the Environmental Protection Agency reports levels are low enough that atrazine probably won't cause reproductive problems. This statement has been criticized, however, and its safety is currently controversial. Tyrone B. Hayes from the University of California at Berkeley (2003) looked at the effect of atrazine on frogs. With increasing exposure to atrazine, some of the frogs began to show both male and female sex organs.

4. **Benzophenone** – A well-known UV filter, this substance is used in the printing industry and in sunscreens. It is also used in perfumes and soaps to prevent UV light from damaging their colors and scents. A study by Kunisue et al. (2012) examined some benzophenone derivatives and their role in endometriosis. The group looked at five benzophenone derivatives in the urine of 625 women in Utah and California. 600 of these women had undergone a laparoscopy, laparotomy or pelvic MRI for a possible endometriosis between 2007 and 2009. Adjusted odds ratios were calculated for benzophenone derivative urinary concentrations and the odds of an endometriosis diagnosis. They were able to find an association between endometriosis and one specific benzophenone derivative – 2,4 OH-BP (2,4 – dihydroxybenzophenone). Several studies have already pointed to the potent xenoestrogen activity of 2,4-OH-BP. One such study was performed by Morohoshi et al. in 2005. This group was able to demonstrate estrogenic activity of several benzophenone derivatives. According to the authors, "Eleven compounds, most of which were benzophenone derivatives and parabens, showed binding affinity to ER [estrogen receptor] by ER-ELISA without s9 mix" (Morohoshi et al., 2005). According to Kunisue et al. (2012), "In vitro studies using recombinant yeast cells that express human ERα [estrogen receptor α] with the β-galactosidase reporter gene demonstrated an

approximate 5-fold higher estrogenic activity of 2,4-OH-BP than bisphenol A (BPA), which is a well-known EDC [endocrine disrupting chemical]" (Kunisue et al., 2012, Benzone Derivatives in Urine and their association with endometriosis section).

5. **Bisphenol A (BPA)** – BPA is a substance that is used to make epoxy and plastic resins. The major exposure route in humans in through the diet, and it is known to be an endocrine disruptor. BPAs can be found in numerous products such as CDs, DVDs, food and beverage cans, sales receipts (thermal paper), sports equipment, water bottles and water pipes. In 2013, the Food and Drug Administration reported that BPA is safe at low levels; however, as of 2014, debates persist on its safety. BPA has been banned for use in baby bottles in Canada and Europe. In addition to being an endocrine disruptor, BPAs may play a role in abnormal thyroid function, cancer, diabetes, heart disease, neurological problems, obesity and reproductive problems.

6. **Butylated hydroxy anisole (BHA)** – Butylated hydroxy anisole is a petroleum by-product that acts as an antioxidant and is used as a food preservative. Specifically, it prevents fats from becoming rancid. It can be found in animal food, cosmetics, medications and rubber. BHA is known to be present in ice cream, shortening, candy, dry cereal, crackers, seasonings and instant potatoes. The National Institutes of Health report BHA is reasonably anticipated to be carcinogenic due to outcomes of some animal studies; however, in humans, the low intakes don't appear to show an increased risk. This chemical may possibly irritate the liver, and some people may be allergic to it.

7. **Dichlorobenzene** – This chemical is a pesticide, deodorant and disinfectant and is probably carcinogenic.

Dichlorobenzene is not easily broken down and can build up in fatty tissues in the human body. In addition, 1,3-dichlorobenzene has been found to have adverse effects on the thyroid and pituitary glands. Exposure comes from breathing the air where it is present. This chemical can be found in mothballs and in toilet deodorizer blocks.

8. **Dichlorodiphenyltrichloroethane (DDT)** – DDT is an insecticide that is classified as "moderately toxic". Its use was banned in 1972. Dichlorodiphenyltrichloroethane is a known endocrine disruptor and has been linked to menstrual disorders and other reproductive problems. Studies have also linked it to several types of cancer. A study done by toxicologist Michael Fry at the University of California at Davis (1995) found female cells in the reproductive tracts of male gulls after they were injected with DDT, DDE and methoxychlor (all xenoestrogens). Although banned, DDT can persist in the soil for centuries.

9. **Dieldrin** – Dieldrin is an insecticide that was used from the 1950s to the 1970s as an alternative to DDT. Specifically, farmers used this chemical to kill pests on crops, and it was used in homes to kill termites. It does not easily break down, and it is toxic to both humans and animals. Dieldrin can be found today in the soil. Plants can absorb it, and it can be found in the fat of animals. In addition to dieldrin being a probable carcinogen, it has been linked to reproductive disorders, breast cancer and Parkinson's disease. It is banned from use in most parts of the world. Those at highest risk are people who live in old homes where this chemical was used to treat termites in the past or those who live near a hazardous waste site.

10. **Endosulfan** – Endosulfan is an insecticide that treats infestations of whiteflies, aphids and leafhoppers. It is

one of the most toxic pesticides known to man, and its use is being discontinued on a global scale. Currently, in the U.S., endosulfan cannot be used in residential homes. The levels of this chemical are regularly monitored in the U.S. by state and federal agencies. In addition to being neurotoxic to both humans and animals, it is an endocrine disruptor. According to The Agency for Toxic Substances and Disease Registry, "Two studies of environmental exposure of humans suggested that endosulfan may be associated with alterations in the levels of thyroid hormones and some sex hormones in the blood." However, they also state that in these studies, participants were also exposed to other pesticides, so it cannot be determined if endosulfan was entirely responsible for these hormonal effects. Most exposure comes by way of diet.

11. **Erythrosine (FD&C Red #3)** – Erythrosine is food coloring agent and is a possible carcinogen. The Center for Science in the Public Interest has petitioned the U.S. FDA to impose a complete ban of erythrosine, but no action has been taken to date.

12. **Ethinyl estradiol** – Ethinyl estradiol is the estrogen component of birth control pills. It is released into the environment as a xenoestrogen through the urine and feces of women who take these pills.

13. **Hepatachlor** – This chemical is an insecticide that smells like camphor. It was used in homes, buildings and on food crops. It has not been used for these purposes since 1988, but it can stick to soil and persist in the environment for decades. It is still cleared for use to kill fire ants in underground power transformers, but it is not clear if it is still being used for that purpose.

Hepatachlor can be found in breast milk, dairy products, drinking water, fish, shellfish, poultry and meat. In addition to being a possible carcinogen, hepatachlor may have a negative impact on fertility and the nervous system. Animal studies have shown that high exposure can cause liver damage and a decrease in fertility.

14. **Gamma-hexachlorocyclohexane (Lindane)** – Lindane is an organochlorine pesticide (OCP) that has been used on humans as a treatment for lice and scabies. (β-hexachlorocyclohexane(β-HCH) is a by-product of lindane and has been shown to be a possible endocrine disruptor and carcinogen. Interestingly, a study done in 2013 showed an increased risk of endometriosis in women who were found to have high blood serum levels of β-HCH (Upson et al., 2013). The women with the highest levels of β-HCH in their blood serum were thirty to seventy percent more likely to have endometriosis than the women with the lowest levels of this chemical in their serum. In addition, in the same study, the researchers found a slight link between another OCP called Mirex and endometriosis. Mirex was used in the 1960s and 1970s as an insecticide against fire ants. Lindane was banned from use in 2009 except for use as a last resort in the treatment of lice and scabies. However, because Lindane and Mirex are stable and persist in the environment, these two chemicals are still of concern today. The researchers concluded "extensive past use of environmentally persistent OCPs in the Unites States or present use in other countries may affect the health of reproductive-age women" (Upson et al., 2013, Abstract).

15. **Metalloestrogens** – These substances have an affinity for estrogen receptors and are therefore possible endocrine disruptors. They also potentially play a role in breast cancer. The following are known metalloestrogens:

Aluminum
Antimony
Arsenite
Barium
Cadmium
Cobalt
Copper
Lead
Mercury
Nickel
Selenite
Tin
Vanadate

16. **Methoxychlor** – Methoxychlor is an insecticide that was used as an alternative to DDT. It was used against all kinds of insects including mosquitos, flies and cockroaches. This chemical was used on agricultural crops and animal feed. It is known to stick to soil; however, it does not appear to build up in the food chain because it is broken down fairly easily in fish and animals. Methoxychlor is not usually found in food or water, and exposure is more likely to occur in those living near a hazardous waste site.

According to the Agency for Toxic Substances and Disease Registry in the U.S. (ATSDR), "Studies in animals show that exposure to methoxychlor adversely affects the ovaries, uterus and mating cycles in females..." They also note that fertility is also decreased with exposure to this chemical. It is a known endocrine disruptor, and it is banned from use.

17. **Parabens** – Parabens are preservatives used in cosmetics and other pharmaceutical products such as makeup, moisturizers, shampoos, shaving cream and toothpaste.

These chemicals are used in cosmetics because they do not cause irritation or allergy. Parabens are also used in baked goods, artificial sweeteners and diet foods. They have weak estrogen activity and have been linked to early menarche in young girls.

18. **Pentachlorophenol** – This chemical is a pesticide and a disinfectant. It is used in wood preservation, paper mills and masonry. Pentachlorophenol can be found in leather and rope, and the EPA reports it is probably carcinogenic. It is rapidly metabolized, so buildup in the environment is probably not a big issue. Today this chemical is primarily used on utility poles and railroad ties, and it is treated as regulated hazardous waste in the United States.

19. **Phenosulfonphthalein (Phenol red)** – This chemical is a red dye that is used in laboratory media as a pH indicator. Phenol red is also found in some home swimming pool test kits. It is a known weak endocrine disruptor.

20. **Polybrominated biphenyls (PBBs)** – Polybrominated biphenyls are used as flame retardants. They were used in electrical products, plastic foam, rugs, textiles and upholstery. Manufacturing of PBBs stopped in 1976 in the U.S.; However, these chemicals don't break down easily in the environment and tend to accumulate. Exposure usually comes from eating contaminated food or living near hazardous waste sites.

PPBs are possible menstruation disruptors. In one study, young girls who were exposed to high levels of PBBs were shown to start menstruating at an earlier age.

21. **Polychlorinated biphenyls (PCBs)** – Polychlorinated biphenyls are used in coolant fluids to help reduce the chance of fire in electrical fields. These chemicals do not

readily decompose and can therefore build up in the environment. They are carcinogenic and have been banned from use since 1979. They were used in carbonless copy paper, caulk, cements, hydraulic fluids, lubricating oils, paints and pesticides. They are known endocrine and nervous system disruptors. PCBs imitate and inhibit estradiol in the human body which may lead to all kinds of menstrual and reproductive disorders and cancers.

22. **Propyl gallate** – This synthetic chemical is an antioxidant added to fats and vegetable oils as a preservative. Specifically, it protects against rancidity by preventing oxidation. It can be found in non-food items such as adhesives, bath products, cosmetics, hair care products, lubricants, sunscreen and toothpaste. Propyl gallate can also be found in foods such as microwavable popcorn, cereal, chewing gum and soups.

23. **Phthalates** – Phthalates are chemicals that are added to plastics to increase flexibility (plasticizer). DEHP, or di(2-ethylhexyl) phthalate, is one phthalate that can leach from hospital IV bags. The FDA has warned that prolonged treatment with IV fluid bags may affect testicular development in young males. Phthalates have been shown to be endocrine disruptors in studies in rats. According to a study by Moore, Rudy, Lin, Ko and Peterson (2001), the phthalate DEHP affects the development of the male reproductive system in rats and caused severe reproductive toxicity in five out of eight litters. Phthalates can be found in adhesives, building supplies, butter, caulk, children's toys, detergents, eye shadow, food containers, floor tiles, hair spray, meats, medication, milk, nail polish, nutritional supplements, packaging materials, paints, printing ink, shower curtains and upholstery. Europe and the Unites States have restricted the use of phthalates in children's toys.

24. **Sodium lauryl sulfate (SLS)** – This chemical is a surfactant that causes cleaning items to foam. SLS is quite often contaminated with the dangerous chemical 1,4-dioxane. The FDA recommends limits on 1,4-dioxane content in cosmetics but has not established a specific limit. Sodium lauryl sulfate can be found in bubble baths, cleaning products, some food products, laundry detergents, pesticides, shampoo, shaving cream and toothpaste. It can be irritating to the eyes, skin and respiratory tract, and prolonged exposure may cause dermatitis. SLS is possibly carcinogenic.

25. **Triclosan** – This chemical is an antibacterial and antifungal agent that is often used in hospitals, and it is especially useful when dealing with patients with MRSA infections (methicillin-resistant staphylococcus aureus). Its safety is under review in both the United States and Canada. Studies have shown that excessive exposure to triclosan may cause a reduction in thyroid hormone levels.

Triclosan can be found in deodorants, detergents, hospital scrubs, mouthwash, shampoo, soaps, cosmetics and toothpaste. This chemical can also be found in non-food items such as clothing, furniture and toys.

Those are some of the most dangerous xenoestrogens that we may be exposed to today. Even though some have been restricted or banned, they persist in the environment and we can still be exposed to them.

The following is another blog that I wrote in 2016 regarding xenoestrogens and hormones. As you will see, the current "BPA-free" plastics may not be safe:

Chemicals That Interfere with Hormones: Disturbing Findings

I have recently started to work on a new book on endocrine disrupting chemicals, or EDC (also known as xenoestrogens). These chemicals have been implicated in the development of adenomyosis, but they have also been implicated in other reproductive disorders and cancers. I wanted to publish an in-depth review of these dangerous chemicals, but little did I know that I would be embarking on a huge project that is also quite disturbing.

I like to use PubMed through the NIH to get reliable information from actual clinical studies. The first study I read was "Mixtures of xenoestrogens disrupt estradiol-induced non-genomic signaling and downstream functions in pituitary cells" by Rene Viñas and Cheryl S. Watson at the University of Texas (2013).

The first interesting thing I noted is that this group looked at the effect of mixtures of xenoestrogens, not just the effect of one xenoestrogen, on rat cells. This is particularly important since we are not exposed to one xenoestrogen at a time. In fact, we are exposed to hundreds of these dangerous chemicals each day. We are bombarded with them the minute we walk out our front door. This study showed that the cells responded differently when exposed to multiple xenoestrogens at the same time as opposed to a single xenoestrogen.

Although that fact is enlightening, the most disturbing thing I learned from this article is about bisphenol A, or BPA. This xenoestrogen is used to make plastics and epoxy resins, and it can be found in a slew of consumer products. Examples include water bottles, thermal paper (such as sales receipts, cinema tickets, airline tickets), CD's, and DVDs. It is also used extensively to line the inside of food and beverage cans. It is one of the highest volume chemicals made in the world today.

In the last ten years or so, the safety of BPA has come into question. Studies have shown that it is an endocrine-disruptor. In particular, it has been shown to interfere with estrogen receptors. Because of this concern, years of discussion ensued in governmental agencies worldwide leading to a ban of BPA use in the production of baby bottles and other products in children under the age of three. Today, some of these products are listed as "BPA-free".

However, this study from the University of Texas pointed out that many "BPA-free" products now contain BPS, or bisphenol S. BPS is now being used as a substitute for BPA. Shockingly, this study shows that BPS is also an endocrine disruptor as it also interferes with estrogen receptors!! So, according to this study, "BPA-free" is NOT safe. As I continued to do my research, I noticed that a 2011 study by Walsh stated "Almost all commercially available plastic products we sampled, independent of the type of resin, product, or retail source, leached chemicals having reliably-detectable EA [endocrine activity], including those advertised as BPA-free. In some cases, BPA-free products released chemicals having more EA that BPA-containing products."

I was stunned! Next, I read a very long and excellent article on Wikipedia about Bisphenol A. I concluded that this chemical hasn't been banned altogether because of lobbyists/politics. Here are some interesting (and infuriating) facts:

1. *The FDA considers BPA to be "safe at the current levels occurring in foods." They base this statement on two studies funded by the chemical companies even though there are hundreds of other studies out*

there that show this chemical to be an endocrine disruptor.

2. The FDA had previously stated that the benefits of good nutrition outweigh the risks of BPA exposure when it comes to infant formulas/food. Since that time, BPA has been banned in baby bottles in the U.S.

3. In 2011, the governor of Maine, Paul LePage, actually made the following statement when discussing the issue of bisphenol A: "The only thing that I've heard is if you take a plastic bottle and put it in the microwave and you heat it up, it gives off a chemical similar to estrogen. So, the worst case is some women may have little beards." In April of that year, the Maine legislature passed a bill that banned the use of BPA in baby bottles and some reusable food containers. Governor LePage refused to sign it.

4. In 2009, the EPA planned on labeling BPA as a "chemical of concern"; however, after lobbyists for the chemical company met with members of the administration, this didn't happen.

This is just the tip of the iceberg. I will get into much more detail in my upcoming book, but I felt the need to write a short blog on this topic now as to alert the public about safety issues regarding BPA and so-called "BPA-free" products. After reading these articles, I have learned that virtually no plastic product is safe, regardless of what the government tells you.

The best advice I can give is to get away from processed food and go as fresh as possible. Organic is best. Try to stay away from canned foods as much as possible. It is important to note that we cannot avoid all xenoestrogens, but it is vitally important to reduce exposure as much as possible. This is particularly important for women who already suffer from estrogen-

dependent disorders such as adenomyosis, endometriosis, and reproductive cancers.

Xenoestrogens are known endocrine disruptors that have been shown many times to affect the functioning of the reproductive tract in both males and females. Although not all scientists and doctors agree on the toxicity of these substances, it would be a good idea to reduce exposure as much as possible. Especially in women who suffer from adenomyosis. According to Slomczynska in an article in the Polish Journal of Veterinary Science (2008), "there is a need for the studies on all potential xenoestrogens to describe tissue-specific activities, and via which pathways in those tissues these compounds will disrupt or mimic hormone action" (Abstract).

Chapter 15 - Synthetic Progesterone vs. Natural Progesterone

"I think that in all the lectures and workshops I give, the question that's asked of me most often is, 'What else can I take besides estrogen?'"

-Dr. Fredi Kronenberg

Synthetic progesterone and natural progesterone are not the same thing. It is important to know the differences between the two as natural progesterone is generally the preferred form to use when trying to balance hormone levels.

The herb called wild yam is the source of a substance called diosgenin. This substance is found naturally in this plant, and it can also be found in soy. Disogenin was extracted from wild yam in the 1930s by a Pennsylvania State College chemistry professor by the name of Russell Marker, and he found that disogenin could be transformed into a biologically active form of progesterone through a chemical process in the laboratory. The progesterone that resulted from this process was biologically identical to the progesterone that was made in our own bodies. However, this discovery also led to the development of a synthetic form of progesterone, also known as a progestin or a progestogen, which is used in the birth control pill. The progesterone in the birth control pill is not bioidentical progesterone.

It is important to note that the diosgenin in wild yam must be converted into bioidentical progesterone in the laboratory. The body cannot make bioidentical progesterone just by consuming wild yam. This will be discussed in further detail later in this chapter.

Drug companies alter natural, bioidentical progesterone so they can patent progestins. Natural substances are not allowed to be patented. So, the drug companies promote the use of progestins because it is good for their bottom line. From a health perspective, however, bioidentical progesterone is the healthy way to go. Examples of progestins include Provera, Megace and Aygestin.

Since progestins are not chemically the same as our own progesterone, they will not have the same activity as our own progesterone. In addition, these substances will also have side effects that will not occur when using natural, bioidentical progesterone.

Side Effects of Progestins (Synthetic Progesterone)

- Breast tenderness
- Weight gain
- Acne
- Insomnia
- Irritability
- Depression
- Spotting
- Bloating
- Low sex drive
- Nausea
- Fatigue
- Headaches including migraines
- Partial vision loss
- Asthma

According to Pamela Smith (2010), "An article in the Journal of the American Medical Association discussed that the risk of developing breast cancer was predicted to rise by nearly 80 percent after ten years of using estrogen and/or progestin (synthetic) HRT [hormone replacement therapy]." Dr. Stephen Sinatra (2001), states "I have found that synthetic progestins can lead to serious cardiac side effects in my patients, including shortness of breath, fatigue, chest pain and high blood pressure".

Benefits of natural progesterone:

- Helps to balance hormone levels, especially in estrogen dominant women
- Has a calming effect – helps with anxiety and mood swings
- Promotes restful sleep
- Diuretic – helps maintain water balance which reduces bloating
- Anti-inflammatory
- Improves sex drive
- Stimulates bone growth
- Lowers cholesterol
- Helps to prevent premenstrual migraine headaches

The most effective way to get natural, bioidentical progesterone into your body is through transdermal application. Progesterone cream is absorbed rapidly through the skin and reaches peak levels in 3 to 4 hours.

Many different progesterone creams are available on the market today. However, not all progesterone creams are created equal. In fact, some of these creams have very little bioidentical progesterone in them. The first and most important thing to know is that just because a product contains "wild yam extract" does not necessarily mean that it contains progesterone. Studies have shown that wild yam cannot be converted into progesterone in the body. Therefore, it is imperative to know if the diosgenin has been converted into an active form of progesterone; otherwise the product is useless. Second, even if an active form of progesterone is available in the cream, it still may have very small amounts in it. Look for the specific amount of progesterone that the cream contains on the label. If it is not on the label, call the company and ask for the dosage amounts. Third, the progesterone needs to be suspended in the proper medium for it to be effectively absorbed. According to Lee and Hopkins (2004), "Products containing mineral oil or wax may prevent the progesterone from being absorbed into the skin."

It is important to note that when progesterone levels are tested in blood serum, as most hormone testing is done, the levels refer mostly to progesterone that is protein-bound which is biologically inactive. When progesterone is processed in the liver, it becomes bound to protein which then allows it to enter the blood serum; however, this form of progesterone does not bind with progesterone receptors because of the presence of the protein attached to it. Therefore, it is inactive. In fact, Dr. John Lee and Virginia Hopkins (2004) state, "When serum or plasma is used in blood tests, more than 90 percent of the progesterone found is protein-bound and no longer bioavailable..." (p. 354-355). This protein-bound progesterone that is picked up by blood serum hormone testing does not represent true biologically-active progesterone.

High-quality progesterone creams that have bioidentical and bioactive progesterone can get past this problem. Progesterone is absorbed well through the skin and is not protein-bound, so it is biologically active and can attach effectively to progesterone receptors. According to Lee and Hopkins (2004), "It begins circulating in the blood within seconds of application and reaches its peak in about 3 to 4 hours. After about 8 hours, levels begin dropping, and most of the progesterone is cleared from the body within 12 hours of application." (p. 355).

Lee and Hopkins recommend that women with estrogen dominance use a progesterone cream that has 400 mg. of bioidentical progesterone per ounce. Some creams have as low as 10 mg. per ounce, and these creams won't work. Also, make sure that it contains progesterone and not just a "wild yam extract". It is also recommended that you rotate the sites of application. Using the same area may saturate the area and reduce the effectiveness of the progesterone. Use in areas where there is good capillary supply and where the skin is thin. Good areas include the inner arms, neck, abdomen, upper chest, palms of hands and breasts. Also, the progesterone is more effectively absorbed when spread on a large area. Dr. David Zava recommends using two doses – one in the morning and one at bedtime – to imitate what your body would do. Use a smaller dose in the morning and a larger dose at bedtime since progesterone has a calming effect and can help you sleep.

Lee and Hopkins (2006) give some great recommendations about hormone balance in their book, "*Dr. John Lee's Hormone Balance Made Simple.*" Before diving head first into the use of natural progesterone, I highly advise reading his book. I also highly advise getting your hormone levels tested through saliva testing. As previously discussed, blood and serum levels of progesterone are about 90 percent protein-bound and inactive. However, a more accurate assessment of hormone levels can be ascertained through saliva testing. This test can be done at home without a prescription from a doctor. All you have to do is to spit in a tube and send it to the lab through the mail. According to Dr. David Zava in Lee and Hopkins book (2006):

"...when hormones are delivered through the skin and enter the bloodstream, a much higher percentage are bioavailable. This shows up in tissues such as those in the salivary gland and then in saliva...This is why a daily dose of 15 to 30 mg of progesterone cream results in a very small increase (if at all) on a blood test, but a significant increase in a saliva test."

Some doctors claim that natural progesterone won't protect your uterus like synthetic progestins. A study by Helene Leonetti et al. (2003) compared the use of PremPro (synthetic estrogen and progesterone) and Premarin (synthetic estrogen) and natural progesterone cream. She found that the women that used the bioidentical progesterone cream were protected against endometrial cancer.

It is possible to overdose on progesterone cream. Therefore, it is so important to monitor your hormone levels and to apply the progesterone cream exactly as recommended. It is also recommended that you use progesterone cream only – not cream combined with other hormones such as estrogen and testosterone.

Warning signs that you have used too much progesterone:

- Sleepiness – most women report feeling very calm.
- Yeast infection
- Depression
- Bloating
- Low sex drive
- Symptoms of estrogen deficiency

Since progesterone is the precursor to all other steroid hormones, some are afraid that the levels of all other steroid hormones will increase as a result of using progesterone cream. This is not the case. It has been found that progesterone applied transdermally will not increase the levels of other hormones. The reason is probably the fact that the cream is absorbed through fat and into the bloodstream (bypassing the ovaries and adrenals). The conversion of progesterone to other hormones occur in the ovaries and adrenal glands.

Lee and Hopkins (2006) state that the use of progesterone cream may specifically help women with endometriosis. According to the authors, "transdermal progesterone can be given in doses similar to that of early pregnancy, starting at day 8 and continuing until day 26 of a usual 28-day cycle. Experience shows that this treatment is often effective in relieving the symptoms of endometriosis." However, they caution that it may take up to six months to see improvement.

The following are a list of natural progesterone creams available on the market today. However, please do your research. When ordering the cream, ask detailed questions:

1. Does the cream have at least 400 mg. progesterone per ounce?
2. Does the cream contain bioidentical estrogen or a "wild yam extract"?
3. What kind of medium is the progesterone suspended in? Does it contain mineral oil or wax?

Please note: I do not promote any of these progesterone creams. It is up to the consumer to research each of these creams prior to purchase to make sure the cream is of high quality.

Restore Natural Progesterone Cream – this cream has 480 mg. progesterone per ounce. It also has no added estrogenic ingredients.

Available through:

Alternative Medicine Network

601 16th Street., #C-#105

Golden, CO 80401

Renewed Balance Progesterone Cream – this cream contains 550 mg. progesterone per ounce. It also has no artificial ingredients and is suspended in vitamin E.

Available through:

AIM International, Inc.

3904 East Flamingo Ave.

Nampa, ID 83687

Dr. Randolph's Natural Progesterone Cream – this cream contains no chemicals and the progesterone is suspended in an excellent liposome delivery formula.

For more information, please visit or call:

www.hormonewell.com

(856)628-6337

Emerita, Pro-Gest – this cream was the first ever progesterone cream. It contains 450 mg. progesterone per ounce, and I have found it in Whole Foods stores. On their website, they explain that they use the Mexican wild yam plant and convert it into bioidentical progesterone in the lab.

621 SW Alder

Suite 900

Portland, OR 97205-3627

Fem-Gest – this cream contains 480 mg. progesterone per ounce. It also contains no artificial dyes or parabens.
Available through:
Bio-Nutritional Formulas
106 East Jericho Turnpike
P.O. Box 311
Mineola, NY 11501

PureGest Lotion – this cream contains about 700 mg. progesterone per ounce. It also contains no mineral oil, parabens, artificial colors or preservatives.
Available through:
Kevala
42 Digital Drive #7
Novato, CA 94949
www.kevalahealth.com

Chapter 16 - How Can Hormonal Balance Be Achieved?

"The food you eat can be either the safest and most powerful form of medicine or the slowest form of poison."

-Ann Wigmore

As I am sure you have concluded, hormonal balance may not necessarily be achieved by simply supplementing with one hormone. All the hormones must be at proper levels since they all interact with each other. The sex hormones interact with cortisol, insulin and thyroid hormones. In addition, other factors play a role in hormonal balance such as stress, toxins (xenoestrogens), an unhealthy diet, medications, and vitamin deficiencies and/or excesses.

The following is a list of suggestions that may help to achieve hormone balance. Women with adenomyosis may see a significant reduction of their symptoms by taking steps to get their hormones in balance.

1. Take a high-quality multivitamin and mineral supplement to ensure you are getting the proper basic nutrients.
2. Educate yourself on how to eat a well-balanced diet that will also promote hormonal balance. See Chapter 17 for more information on this subject.
3. Be sure to get plenty of fiber since estrogen is excreted through the bowel.
4. Include a high-quality omega-3 supplement to your vitamin regime. See Chapter 19 for an in-depth discussion of omega-3 fatty acids.
5. Use a high-quality bioidentical progesterone cream. See Chapter 15 for a list of good progesterone creams.
6. If overweight, make it a goal to lose the excess body fat. Exercise at least three times per week and be sure to include strength training.
7. Reduce your stress level. Get rid of things in your life that aren't necessary and learn to say "no".

8. Consider doing a detoxification cleanse. The liver processes estrogen and eliminates toxins including xenoestrogens. If the liver is sluggish, this may increase the problem of estrogen dominance. A detoxification cleanse is well worth the effort. See Chapter 4 for more information on liver health.
9. Quit smoking.
10. Lower exposure to xenoestrogens. See Chapter 14 for more information on this topic.
11. Be careful with hormone replacement therapy (HRT). Taking unopposed estrogen (estrogen without progesterone) can lead to estrogen dominance and can increase your risk of cancer. Do your research before you decide to go on HRT.
12. Cut down on coffee consumption. Studies have shown women who consume four to five cups of coffee per day have 70% more circulating estrogen in their bodies as compared to those women who consume less than one cup per day (Lam, 2105b).
13. Do not store or heat any food in a plastic container. All food should be stored and/or heated in glass or ceramic containers.
14. Avoid using plastic wrap to store food.
15. Used unbleached paper products.
16. Use natural fragrances such as pure essential oils. DoTerra® is an excellent choice.
17. Use all-natural laundry detergents. Good companies include Seventh Generation®, Green Shield® and The Honest Company®
18. Use all-natural dish detergent. Good companies include Seventh Generation®, Eco-Me® and Whole Foods Market®
19. Use natural herbicides and pesticides. There are many ways to control pests. The following options are easy to prepare:
   A. 1 cup salt to 1 gallon vinegar. Mix and put in a spray bottle.

B. Fill a spray bottle half full of vinegar and finish filling it with all-natural liquid soap.
C. Sprinkle diatomaceous earth around plants.
D. Sprinkle a small amount of eucalyptus oil around plants.
E. Use onion, garlic or cayenne pepper for pest control.
F. For ants, use 1 tbsp. peppermint essential oil in 1 liter of water and put in a spray bottle. Another option is to put 5-10 drops of any citrus essential oil and 1 tsp. cayenne pepper in 1 quart of water. Put in spray bottle.
G. Use ½ tsp. neem, ½ tsp. natural liquid soap, fill to one gallon with water and put into a spray bottle.

20. Use all-natural cleaning products. Seventh Generation®, Green Shield®, Biokleen® and The Honest Company® products are good options.
21. Only buy grass-fed organic meats that say "hormone-free".
22. Avoid salmon that has been farm-raised as it contains high levels of PCBs, pesticides, antibiotics and other drugs. According to Lee and Hopkins (2006), "...salmon farms use more antibiotics by weight than any other farmed animal. Furthermore, their fat is lower in the beneficial essential fatty acids than wild salmon." Look for "wild Pacific" salmon.
23. Buy organic fruits and vegetables. If you do buy non-organic fruits and vegetables, wash thoroughly and peel before eating.
24. Restrict intake of dairy products.
25. Use a high-quality water filter.
26. Although birth control pills are often prescribed for adenomyosis, if possible, try to avoid this treatment. BCPs can deplete the body of copper, zinc, folate, vitamin B6 and vitamin B12. Also, according to Pamela Smith (2010), "women taking birth control pills have been shown to have decreased serum testosterone and DHEA levels." Instead, try using a condom without a spermicide

or a levonorgestrel IUD. These are just things to think about, and each woman will have to make her own decision. The decision on whether to use BCPs or an IUD is a hard one as both options have their positives and negatives.

27. Use bioidentical hormones to treat hormonal imbalances. Check out bioidentical progesterone cream.

28. Use all-natural baby products. Good companies include Babyganics®, The Honest Company® and Baby Earth®.

29. Use natural cosmetics. Good companies include Bare Minerals®, Ecco Bella®, Physicians Formula®, Origins® and Burt's Bees®.

30. Use natural lotions and moisturizers. Good companies include 100% Pure®, Bella Floria®, and Nature's Gate®.

31. Use natural toothpaste. Good companies include Tom's of Maine® and Kiss My Face®.

32. Try to avoid shower curtains. Install a glass shower door if possible.

33. Use a zinc oxide-based sunscreen.

34. Try to avoid canned foods. Frozen is better.

35. If your home is newly painted or carpeted, make sure there is proper ventilation.

36. Avoid plastic water bottles.

37. Use all-natural soaps. Good companies include Dr. Bronner's®, Ballard Organics® and The Honest Company®.

38. Use all-natural shampoos and conditioners. Good companies include Avalon Organics®, Burt's Bees®, Aveda® and The Honest Company®.

39. Try to avoid the fertilizer/pesticide areas in home improvement stores.

40. Turn off the TV and other lights when sleeping. Being exposed to light while sleeping reduces melatonin levels.

41. Throw away nail polish and nail polish remover.

42. Fabric softeners contain petrochemicals which are known xenoestrogens. Don't use if possible.

Section IV

Chapter 17 - Does a Poor Diet Cause Adenomyosis?

"People's idea of the balanced diet has changed from the archaic 'four-food group' approach of meals containing a meat, a dairy food, a cereal grain and fruits and vegetables to a more natural diet, lower in fat protein and refined carbohydrates."

-Dr. Elson Haas

Studies have shown that estrogen levels are lower in women who consume a low-fat, high-fiber diet in comparison to women who consume a high-fat diet full of processed food. This clearly shows that proper diet is of utmost importance in women who suffer from adenomyosis.

According to Elizabeth Lipiski (2000), in the last 10 years, there has been a 10 percent decrease in the amount of vegetables consumed and a 60 percent increase in the number of soft drinks consumed. Other researchers have reported that 60 percent of calories from today's diet come from refined sugars and fat. Food processing has also led to nutritional problems. Rudin and Felix, in their book "Omega-3 Oils: A Practical Guide", states "As food processing techniques removed the vitamins, fiber and other essential nutrients from our foods, the modern maladies grew rampant." For these reasons, it is important to focus on diet and improve it to reduce adenomyosis symptoms.

Foods contain proteins, carbohydrates, fats and/or fiber. Carbon, hydrogen and oxygen are obtained from the intake of any of these types of foods, but nitrogen can only be obtained from protein. These elements are necessary for the functioning of the body at the cellular level.

Twenty percent of our body weight comes from protein. Proteins are derived from foods such as meat, milk, eggs and fish and are broken down into amino acids in the body. Eight of these are essential meaning that they must be obtained from the diet.

These amino acids are stored in the liver and are used to manufacture glucagon. Glucagon, in turn, is involved in the release of glycogen which is a source of energy for the body. Proteins are important in the development of skin, teeth and bones. In addition, they build and repair damaged tissue and are

The Eight Essential Amino Acids

- Isoleucine
- Leucine
- Lysine
- Methionine
- Phenylalanine
- Threonine
- Tryptophan
- Valine

important in enzyme and hormone production. Proteins are broken down by gastric juices and are difficult to digest since they use more energy in the digestion process than do other types of food. Deep frying and charbroiling make them even more difficult to digest. The typical American eats two to ten times the amount of protein than they actually need. Too much protein in the diet puts a strain on the kidneys resulting in damaged renal tubules and decreased kidney function. It also forces the kidneys to excrete excess calcium.

Proteins come in two forms: complete and incomplete. Complete proteins are those that contain all eight essential amino acids: tryptophan (a precursor to serotonin), lysine, methionine, phenylalanine, threonine, valine, leucine and isoleucine. These are present in animal products such as poultry, beef, pork, milk and eggs. Incomplete proteins are those that do not have all eight essential amino acids present but can be combined to form a complete protein. Plant foods are sources of incomplete proteins. An example of food combining that results in a complete protein is rice and beans.

Carbohydrates supply us with a steady supply of energy throughout the day. Four calories (a unit of energy) are produced for each gram of carbohydrate consumed. Complex carbohydrates are better than the simple carbohydrates and are a rich source of fiber, vitamins and minerals. Also, carbohydrates work alongside protein and fats to help support the immune system and keep joints healthy. Therefore, it is so important to never completely eliminate carbohydrates when dieting.

Carbohydrates are broken down quickly into mono-, di- or poly-saccharides. Monosaccharides are simple sugars that are absorbed by the body without changing form. Examples include glucose and fructose. The disaccharides are broken down partially by the enzymes in saliva. Examples include lactose, sucrose (table sugar) and maltose. The polysaccharides (also known as starches) are derived from complex carbohydrates and require amylase or other catalysts for digestion. The digestion is completed in the small intestine where they pass into the blood and are used by cells for energy. Examples of polysaccharides include wheat, rice, corn, legumes, and vegetables. Any unused energy is stored in the liver as glycogen. When the body needs energy, the glycogen is converted back to glucose by the liver.

An important component of complex carbohydrates is fiber. This important food is found in the skins of fruits and vegetables and in the outer covering of wheat (wheat bran). Fiber is indigestible material that aids in healthy gastrointestinal function and elimination as it stimulates peristalsis. Fiber does not produce calories and therefore does not produce any energy. Cellulose and hemicellulose are two major forms of fiber, both of which absorb water and create bulk. If the diet is high in fiber but low in water consumption, constipation may result, so it is extremely important to drink plenty of water especially if taking a fiber supplement.

Fats are found in foods such as butter, lard, bacon and oils and are broken down in the body into fatty acids. They are easy to digest and a great source of quick energy. Fats, including the extremely important omega-3 fatty acids, are discussed in detail in chapter 19.

I want to urge you to consider natural and organic foods as much as possible, especially foods that are grown locally. Try to purchase foods at local farmer's markets if possible. The reason for this is that the fresher the food, the more nutrients that are available for your body to use. Also, foods in supermarkets are usually loaded with pesticides and herbicides that are known to be endocrine disruptors. This topic is discussed at length in Chapter 14.

The following is a list of produce sold in supermarkets that contain the highest amounts of pesticides (Lam, 2015a):

Apples
Apricots
Bell peppers
Peaches
Spinach
Strawberries

The following is a list of produce sole in supermarkets that contain the least amounts of pesticides (Lam, 2015a):

Avocados
Bananas
Broccoli
Cauliflower
Corn

Green onions
Onions
Sweet potatoes

Keep this in mind when referring to the following recommended foods to help treat adenomyosis and estrogen dominance. If you do not have access to natural/organic foods, it is recommended that you wash fresh produce thoroughly before consuming.

1. **Cruciferous vegetables** – These vegetables contain a substance called indole-3-carbinol (I3C) which is known to help detoxify the liver. I3C also helps the body to inactivate estradiol and balance hormone levels. WebMD (2016) reports it is "possibly effective" against cervical dysplasia. However, I3C is also known to interact with certain medications. Avoid excessive consumption in pregnancy. Also, these specific foods are known to increase intestinal gas, so increase your consumption slowly to let your body adjust. The following list contains some of the more commonly found cruciferous vegetables: arugula, broccoli, bok choy, brussel sprouts, cabbage, cauliflower, collard greens, kale, mustard greens, radish, rutabaga, turnip and watercress.

2. **Mushrooms** – Mushrooms interfere with the production of aromatase which in turn can lower estrogen levels making them an optimum food for those suffering from estrogen dominance. Shiitake and Portobello are the best types to use for this purpose.

3. **Fiber** – This nutrient is of utmost importance in those suffering from adenomyosis. It helps rid the body of excess estrogen by regulating bowel function. By feeding the normal flora (good bacteria) in the gastrointestinal tract, fiber helps to metabolize hormones. It binds to estrogen and helps to eliminate it from the body through the bowel. An intake of at least fifteen grams per day

should be the goal. Increase your fiber intake slowly as it may cause excessive gas. In addition, make sure to drink plenty of water. Taking fiber without drinking enough water could cause constipation.

RDA = 25 g. per day for women.

The following list contains foods high in fiber: fruits (especially prunes, raisins, pears and raspberries), nuts (especially walnuts, almonds, pecans and peanuts), legumes (especially split peas, navy beans, kidney beans and pinto beans), whole grains (especially shredded wheat, oatmeal, whole wheat spaghetti and oatmeal), fresh vegetables (especially artichokes, squash and turnip greens), rye and/or wheat bread and seeds.

4. **Foods high in sulfur** – Sulfur is present in the body as a part of 4 amino acids: methionine, cystine, cysteine and taurine. These amino acids are involved in the production of biotin, coenzyme A, lipoic acid and glutathione, so in essence, sulfur is necessary to keep the liver functioning optimally. This helps the body to rid itself of excess estrogen efficiently.

    RDA = none, but 850 mg. is generally thought to be optimal.

    The following are foods that are high in sulfur: bananas, beef, Brussel sprouts, cabbage, chicken, chives, coconut, cruciferous vegetables, egg yolks, fish, garlic, leeks, pineapple, onions, turnips and watermelon.

5. **Foods high in magnesium** – Magnesium is an extremely important mineral involved in over 100 enzymatic reactions and is known as a natural tranquilizer because of its ability to relax muscles. In fact, taking a calcium and

magnesium supplement together at bedtime may aid in more restful sleep.

Sixty-five percent of magnesium is found in the bones and teeth. Caffeine, alcohol, diuretics and sugar have been shown to decrease levels of magnesium in the body. It is absorbed best if taken on an empty stomach along with vitamin C.

Foods high in magnesium may help increase progesterone production which may help with estrogen dominance. Magnesium may help with bloating, anxiety, depression, fatigue, insomnia, PMS and breast pain. To treat these symptoms, it is best to take magnesium with vitamin B6.

RDA = 400 mg. for non-pregnant women, 18-49 years of age.

The following foods contain good amounts of magnesium: almonds, avocado, black beans, bran, Brazil nuts, brown rice, cashews, dark chocolate, edamame, figs, flaxseed, kale, kidney beans, lentils, mackerel, molasses, oatmeal, peanuts, pumpkin, quinoa, roast beef, sesame seeds, spinach, squash, sunflower seeds, swiss chard and whole wheat bread.

6. **Foods high in zinc** – This mineral is known to be a necessary component of more than 100 enzymes. In addition to its well-known role in the maintenance of the immune system, it is also known to play a role in the maintenance of sexual function. Iron, copper, lead and cadmium are known to compete with zinc for absorption.

    According to Haas (1992), zinc is found in the outer part of grain while cadmium, a toxic heavy metal (see Chapter 14), commonly contaminates the inner part of the grain.

Therefore, refined grains in which the outer covering has been removed, may result in a higher intake of cadmium and a lower intake of zinc. This may lead to possible heavy metal poisoning and a deficiency of zinc, so again, it is important to eat natural, organic whole grains instead of refined food products.

This nutrient supports the breakdown and elimination of estrogen by helping to improve liver function. It is part of a substance called alcohol dehydrogenase which helps the liver to detoxify several different kinds of alcohol. Zinc has also been shown to be low in women with menstrual abnormalities and PMS. In addition, birth control pills are known to reduce zinc levels which in turn raises copper levels. These low zinc levels coupled with high copper levels and low vitamin B6 may lead to depression.

RDA = 8 mg. for non-pregnant women aged 18-49.

The following foods are high in zinc: baked beans, beef, cashews, chicken, crab, dark chocolate, egg yolks, lamb, lobster, milk products, pine nuts, pork, pumpkin seeds, rye, oats, oysters, sunflower seeds, wheat germ, and whole wheat.

7. **Foods high in omega-3 fatty acids** – These nutrients help the body to balance hormone levels and reduce inflammation. An imbalance of omega-3 to omega-6 fatty acids in the diet has been shown to be a factor in estrogen dominance. A more in-depth discussion of fatty acids is found in Chapter 19. The following are foods high in omega-3 fatty acids: anchovies, canola oil, edamame, flaxseed, halibut, herring, naturally fed beef and dairy products, mackerel, olive oil, oysters, wild salmon, sardines, soybean oil, trout, walnuts, wild rice and winter squash.

8. **Organic foods** – Because of the way they are grown, these foods contain less xenoestrogens thereby decreasing the amount of exposure to these dangerous chemicals.

9. **Foods high in taurine** – An essential amino acid, this substance promotes bile circulation and acts as a diuretic. Since it contains sulfur, taurine aids in liver health and toxin removal from the body. Estradiol decreases the amount of taurine formed in the liver, so those with estrogen dominance should ensure that they eat plenty of food that is high in this amino acid. Avoid use in cases of bipolar disorder since taurine is known to interact with lithium. Good food sources include fish, animal meats, eggs and Brewer's yeast.

10. **Foods high in B vitamins** – these vitamins are known to balance hormone levels and improve liver function. Specifically, they help to break down and eliminate estrogen in the liver. Excess estrogen competes with vitamin B6, so this vitamin may reduce the levels of estradiol in the body. In 1942, a researcher by the name of Biskind found that a vitamin B deficiency allowed for inefficient metabolization of estrogen in the liver. It is also known that B6 is involved in the production of taurine which is necessary for liver health. Overall, evidence for the use of vitamin B6 is fairly strong in cases of PMS, menopause, morning sickness, depression and fibrocystic disease.

RDAs:

Vitamin B1 (thiamine): 1.1 mg. for women over 19
Vitamin B2 (riboflavin): 1.1 mg. for women over 19
Vitamin B6 (pyridoxine): 1.3 mg. for women aged 19-50
Vitamin B12 (cobalamin): 2.4 mcg. for women over 14

Vitamin B3 (niacin): 14 mg. for women over 14
Vitamin B5 (pantothenic acid): 5 mg. women over 14
Vitamin B7 (biotin): 30 mcg. for women over 19
Vitamin B9 (folic acid): 400 mcg. for women over 14

The following list contains foods high in vitamin B complex: avocado, bananas, beans, chicken, eggs, leafy greens, lentils, milk, nuts, pomegranate, potatoes, salmon, tuna, turkey, whole grain cereals and yogurt.

11. **Foods high in vitamin E** – this vitamin helps the body to reduce levels of prostaglandins and helps to balance out the estrogen to progesterone ratio. In addition to being an excellent antioxidant, it is also a blood thinner. Several studies have concluded that vitamin E helps to reduce PMS symptoms. It has also been found to reduce the symptoms of vaginal atrophy and has helped to reduce breast pain.

RDA = 33 IU for non-pregnant women aged 18-49.

The following foods contain high levels of vitamin E: almonds, blueberries, olives, spinach and sunflower seeds.

12. **Resveratrol** – Also known as 3,4',5-trihydroxystilbene, resveratrol is a type of phytoestrogen called a stilbene. The topic of phytoestrogens will be discussed at length in the next chapter. A great source of resveratrol is red grapes, and this is the reason for many of the health benefits of red wine. This compound can also be found in grape juice, blueberries, cranberries and peanuts.

This compound contains proanthocyanidins which are known to help block the production of estrogen. However, studies show that resveratrol can act as both an estrogen agonist and an estrogen antagonist. In fact, the chemical structure of resveratrol is very similar to the estrogen agonist diethylstilbestrol. According to the Linus Pauling Institute at Oregon State University, "In cell culture experiments, resveratrol was found to act either as an estrogen agonist or as an estrogen antagonist depending on such factors as cell type, estrogen receptor isoform (ERα or ERβ), and the presence of endogenous estrogens." A study performed by Mendex da Silva et al. (2017) showed that resveratrol, although sometimes used as a treatment for endometriosis, was not found to be superior to placebo. Another study by Gehn, McAndrews, Chien and Jameson (1997) concluded that "...resveratrol is a phytoestrogen and that it exhibits variable degrees of estrogen receptor agonism in different tests systems." Because of the results of these studies, it is generally recommended to avoid the use of this supplement in cases of estrogen-dependent cancers and disorders. It is advisable to refrain from using resveratrol in adenomyosis and endometriosis until further research is done.

13. **Seaweed** – Nori, kelp and kombu are three types of seaweed that can be eaten as a food. Seaweed contains high amounts of fiber, iodine and calcium. In addition, it contains good amounts of protein, vitamin A, vitamin B12 and omega-3 fatty acids. This food stimulates the production of T-cells which improves the immune system. A good way to get seaweed into your diet is to eat sushi or California vegetable rolls.

14. **Red raspberry leaf tea** – see Chapter 20.

Foods to avoid:

1. **All processed food**

2. **Caffeine** – Schliep et al. (2012) found moderate caffeine consumption reduced estradiol concentrations in Caucasian women. However, intake of caffeinated soda and green tea showed an increase in estradiol concentrations among women of all races. Also, Pamela Smith (2010) states "a study showed that women who consume high amounts of caffeine (5 to 7 grams per month) have a 1.2 times greater risk of developing endometriosis." These results suggest that low to moderate consumption of caffeine is probably best for women with adenomyosis/estrogen dominance.

3. **Coffee** – Although Schliep et al. found moderate caffeine consumption reduced estradiol in white women, a 2015 study by Lam showed that women who drink four to five cups of coffee a day had about seventy percent more estrogen in their body as compared to women who drank less than one cup per day. He also states that drinking too much coffee may lead to adrenal fatigue a lower production of progesterone. So according to these studies, moderation is key.

4. **Refined sugar**

5. **Animal meats** – A diet low in animal meats may reduce inflammation. If you eat meat, try to purchase naturally-fed and hormone-free products.

6. **Alcohol and drugs** – Intake of both alcohol and drugs should be eliminated or kept at a minimum because they impair the liver's detoxification activities.

7. **Foods with high amounts of saturated fat**

8. **Fried foods**

9. **Soft drinks**

10. **Reduce intake of dairy products** – dairy is known to increase inflammation, so reducing your intake of these products may help to overall reduce pain and inflammation associated with adenomyosis.

Chapter 18 - Do Phytoestrogens Help or Worsen Adenomyosis?

"I know of no subject more confused, emotionally charged, and important in our lives than food and nutrition and their influence on our well-being."

-Dr. Andrew Weil, from his book, Eating Well for Optimum Health

This question is a very hard one to answer at the present time due to lack of sufficient scientific studies on the subject. Additionally, there are differing opinions due to different theories that have been developed. In this chapter, I will present all the differing opinions as well as the results of the few scientific studies that have been done. It will be up to the reader to decide if she wants to try to incorporate more phytoestrogens into her diet or try to eliminate some of the more questionable sources. I highly recommend consultation with an expert in diet/nutrition and/or an herbalist for more information before taking these steps to deal with adenomyosis.

The role of phytoestrogens in women with adenomyosis and estrogen dominance is confusing to say the least. There is some disagreement within the natural health care and medical field as to whether phytoestrogens increase estrogen levels or help to combat estrogen dominance. Before I go any further, it is important to understand the basics on how different types of estrogen exert their influence in the human body.

In a woman's body, many different tissues have estrogen receptors. Think of it as a couple of puzzle pieces. When estrogen becomes available, it will fit into one of these puzzle slots (receptor sites). Once in place, through a series of chemical reactions, estrogen will begin to exert its influence on the ovaries, uterus or other organs that are susceptible to its influence.

There are many different types of estrogen. The three that are discussed here are endogenous estrogen, xenoestrogens and phytoestrogens. As previously discussed, endogenous estrogen is made in a woman's body and is produced specifically for the proper functioning of the reproductive tract. Xenoestrogens are dangerous, man-made chemicals that act like estrogens in the body and are many times more powerful than human estrogen. They should be avoided at all costs. In general, most phytoestrogens are found in foods and plants and are much weaker than endogenous estrogen.

Although not all natural health care practitioners are in agreement, many believe that a diet high in phytoestrogens will improve conditions associated with estrogen dominance. The theory is that phytoestrogens will bind up the estrogen receptor sites. Two estrogen receptor sites are currently known – ERα and ERβ. Phytoestrogens bind to both but prefer to bind to ERβ.
Therefore, if a woman is exposed to excess amounts of estradiol and/or xenoestrogens, there would be very few receptors to bind to, so these dangerous estrogens would not be activated within the body. Also, since phytoestrogens are much weaker, the estrogenic effect in a woman's body would be much weaker, thereby reducing the risk of estrogen dominance.

Some studies confirm this theory. A study by Rebbeck et al. (2007) showed the use of the black cohosh (an herb that contains phytoestrogens) in women with breast cancer may have a protective effect. Black cohosh has been used for many years to treat menopausal symptoms, and it is reported to have anti-estrogenic effects. The authors of this study caution it is not clear exactly how black cohosh works, and its activity may not actually be associated with hormonal status.

Another study Bacciottini et al. (2007) report genistein (a phytoestrogen found in soy) has one third of the potency of endogenous estrogen when it binds to ERα and one thousandth of the potency when it binds to ERβ. This would seem to suggest that soy would be a good food to include for women with adenomyosis. However, other studies show that soy should not be used in estrogen-sensitive conditions.

Soy contains the highest level of isoflavones in any food source, and these isoflavones are the strongest form of phytoestrogens known. Patisaul and Jefferson (2010, Section 7.4, para. 2) report that genistein, "alters ovarian differentiation, reduces fertility and causes uterine cancer later in life" in mice studies. They also report genistein alters ovarian function in mice. However, they conclude in their report that "moderation is likely key and the incorporation of real foods, as opposed to supplements or processed foods to which soy protein is added, is probably essential for maximizing health benefits" (Section 9, para. 2).

It is important to understand that each phytoestrogen works differently. Recently studies have been done that show some phytoestrogens are as potent as estradiol. Some help with menopausal symptoms by raising estrogen levels while others, such as black cohosh, are anti-estrogenic.

Zava, Dolbaum and Blen (1998) performed a very detailed study of some of the most common herbs and their interactions with estrogen and progesterone receptors. They identified each herb as an estrogen or progesterone agonist or antagonist. An agonist refers to a substance that binds with a receptor and activates it, and an antagonist refers to a substance that binds to the receptor without exhibiting a biological response. In the case of adenomyosis, herbs that are estrogen antagonists and progesterone agonist are the types of herbs that you would want to use. It is inadvisable to use strong estrogen agonists due to the possibility of worsening estrogen dominance.

Much more research needs to be done to fully understand how phytoestrogens work in the human body. Many factors have not been addressed such as absorption, bioavailability once the food/herb has been ingested, and the effects and interactions of other substances in the food/herb. In addition, the way the herb acts in these studies (in vitro) may not be the way the food/herb acts in the human body (in vivo).

According to Seidl and Stewart (1998, Results section, para. 5), "the relative potency of phytoestrogens is, at most, only 2% that of estradiol." Also, this same group reports the consumption of phytoestrogens are considered safe. However, Zava et al. (1998) showed in their study that some phytoestrogens can be as strong as estradiol.

I had a very interesting discussion with a member of Adenomyosis Fighters about this topic. The topic of liver health came up regarding phytoestrogens. What if a woman with adenomyosis took phytoestrogens to combat estrogen dominance but her liver was unhealthy? This could potentially lead to an exacerbation of estrogen dominance because, even though in theory the phytoestrogens occupied the estrogen receptor sites, the xenoestrogens/endogenous estrogens would remain in her body because her liver would not be able to metabolize them. Then, when the phytoestrogens "unlock" from the receptor sites, the more dangerous estrogens would then lock into them and activate. In this situation, phytoestrogens would just make the problem worse. According to Lee and Hopkins (2004, p. 46), "The longer a synthetic estrogen stays in the body, the more opportunity it has to do damage." Clearly, it is of utmost importance to keep your liver healthy, especially if you decide to try phytoestrogens to combat estrogen dominance.

The following foods are known to be good sources of phytoestrogens:

    Almonds
    Apples
    Barley
    Beans
    Berries

Cabbage
Carrots
Flaxseed
Garlic
Grapes
Lentils
Multigrain bread
Oats
Onion
Pears
Pistachios
Plums
Pomegranate
Rice
Rye bread
Sesame seeds
Spinach
Sprouts
Sunflower seeds
Tea
Wheat
Wine
Yams

As you can see, this topic is quite complicated. Because of discrepancies in the research, it is highly advised that you only use phytoestrogens sparingly and under the supervision of a health care practitioner. If you do decide to use some phytoestrogens, remember to keep your liver healthy. It is extremely important that your body can break down estrogen effectively.

Chapter 19 - Do Essential Fatty Acids Help or Worsen Adenomyosis?

"Fat has become a foul three-letter word in our society. We've become a nation of fat phobics, and some of us try to avoid this nutrient at all costs in an effort to lose weight and improve our health. Yet this war on fat has been completely misguided."

– Barry Sears

Before I get into a discussion of fats, I would like to share a portion of a blog that I wrote on my adenomyosis website:

> *During the time that I dealt with adenomyosis, the non-fat diet fad was quite popular. In my attempt to eat healthy, my ex-husband and I tried to buy as much non-fat food as we could, thinking at the time that this was the right thing to do. Boy, were we ever wrong!! My struggle with adenomyosis was at its worst during the time that I was on this non-fat diet – excruciating abdominal pain, very heavy menstrual bleeding with clots, severe bloating – it was just horrible.*
>
> *After putting up with these monthly symptoms for several years, I read an article about the health benefits of flaxseed. I learned that this food contained high levels of omega-3 fatty acids and was found to be helpful in a slew of medical issues. I was intrigued. After years of different birth control pills, antispasmodics, and pain killers, I was ready to try just about anything.*
>
> *I began to sprinkle ground flaxseed on just about anything I ate – yogurt, spaghetti sauce, salad...even a peanut butter and jelly sandwich. The taste was rather earthy if eaten on its own, but when added it to these dishes, I couldn't really taste it at all.*
>
> *Several months went by, and I noticed a significant decrease in my pain level and heavy bleeding. I still had problems, but it was definitely better than where I had been before I added flaxseed to my diet. This led to more*

research on omega-3s, and I quickly realized that a non-fat diet was, in fact, not healthy. I learned that some fat is necessary for optimum health. At the same time, I learned how the Western diet is overloaded with omega-6 fatty acids while deficient in omega-3s.

Fat is needed for both immediate and reserve energy since it supplies two times as many calories per molecule as compared to carbohydrates or protein. They are also needed to help the body to absorb the fat-soluble vitamins. Additionally, fats are required for nerve insulation and are important in the proper functioning of nerve synapses.

Omega-3 fatty acids fall into the category of essential fatty acids (EFAs). These fatty acids are called "essential" because they cannot be made in the body and must come from the diet. To completely understand the role of omega-3 fatty acids in the human body, it is important to understand the difference between saturated and unsaturated fats.

Made up of hydrogen, carbon and oxygen, fats, also referred to as lipids, are insoluble in water. Ninety-five percent of lipids are triglycerides while the other five percent consist of phospholipids such as lecithin and sterols such as cholesterol.

A saturated fat is one in which every bond of a carbon atom is occupied. Each carbon has four bonds that connect them to H (hydrogen) and O (oxygen). The following is a very simplified example of what a saturated fat would look like:

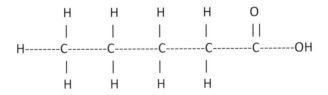

As you can see, each carbon atom is "saturated" – that is, all four of their bonds are occupied. These types of fats are solid at room temperature and are known to increase cholesterol. Examples include butter, meat and lard.

Unsaturated fats are ones in which the carbons are not completely saturated with hydrogen atoms. Since not all carbon atoms are paired, double bonds form between carbons. The more double bonds a fat has, the more unsaturated it is. Below is another very simplified example of what an unsaturated fat would look like:

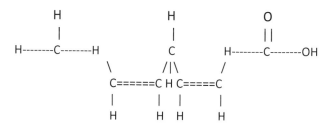

The carbons with the double bonds can accept another hydrogen atom and are therefore unstable and reactive. Also note that the chain is now kinked as opposed to the saturated fat where the chain is straight.

The more bonds between carbons, the more fluid the fat. Since polyunsaturated fats have several missing hydrogens which results in several double bonds between carbons, these types of fats remain liquid at both room temperature and in the refrigerator. These oils have been shown to help prevent heart disease. Examples of polyunsaturated fats include fish oil, corn oil, soybean oil and sunflower oil. Two very important polyunsaturated fats are the long-chained omega-3 and omega-6 fatty acids which are discussed later.

A monounsaturated fat has only two missing hydrogen atoms and therefore only one double bond. They are liquid at room temperature but turn cloudy in the refrigerator. Shown to decrease cholesterol, examples include olive, canola and peanut oil.

There are three categories of fats (lipids): simple, compound and derived. Simple lipids consist of the mono-, di- and tri-glycerides. The mono- and di-glycerides help to make hydrogenated products more pliable. The triglycerides are the major storage form of fatty acids. They consist of one glycerol molecule and three fatty acid molecules. Compound lipids contain a non-lipid part in their composition. Lecithin, glycolipids and lipoproteins are examples of compound lipids. Lipoproteins are surrounded by a protein coating which reacts with water. Therefore, it can easily be transported in the bloodstream. Derived lipids are fatty acids that are related in some way to co-enzyme A. One example is cholesterol.

Fats can be found either in their natural or unnatural forms. Cis fats are in their natural form and are the healthiest fats to consume. The hydrogens of the fatty acid are on the same side of the carbon chain. Since these hydrogens naturally repel each other, the carbon chain will bend away from the hydrogen side. These kinks help the cell to be more fluid and flexible which allows a healthy exchange of nutrients in and out of the cell. Trans fats are the unnatural form of fats and are extremely unhealthy. Since the hydrogen atoms are on the opposite sides of the carbon chain, no bending of the chain takes place and it remains straight. To make trans fats, a hydrogen atom is added to an unsaturated fat through a process called hydrogenation. This procedure is used to prolong the shelf life of the product since unsaturated fats tend to oxidize and turn rancid easily.

Hydrogenated fats are implicated in inflammatory conditions, cancer and heart disease. Some examples of a trans-fat are partially hydrogenated vegetable oil, solid shortenings, hydrogenated lard and solid margarines. These fats contribute to high cholesterol and clogged arteries by infiltrating cell membranes and reacting with enzymes so that fatty acids can't do their job. According to Elizabeth Lipski in her book Digestive Wellness (2000), "European research has shown that essential fatty acids found in the cis formation are necessary for electrical and energy exchanges that involve sulfur-containing proteins, oxygen and light. Trans fatty acids are not suitable in these processes and jam the 'plug' for the cis fats. These electrical currents are responsible for all body functions, from the way our minds work to heartbeat, cell division, muscle coordination and energy levels."

Hydrogenated fats can be found in the spleen, liver, muscles, heart, adrenals and breast milk. They obstruct twenty to forty percent of enzymes and increase the body's need for essential fatty acids. In addition, the process of hydrogenation destroys omega-3 fatty acids leaving those who consume a highly processed diet dangerously deficient in these essential fatty acids.

Fatty acids are stored in the body as triglycerides. They consist of a carbon chain which has a carboxyl group (COOH) attached at the end as shown below:

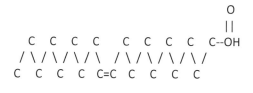

Oleic acid

Fatty acids are usually twelve to twenty-four carbons in length. The function of fatty acids includes maintenance of cell wall integrity, regulation of the metabolism of cholesterol, and regulation of inflammation. They are also precursors to three hormones: prostaglandins, prostacyclins and thromboxanes. As previously discussed, these substances play major roles in the inflammatory process.

The Essential Fatty Acids (EFAs)

These fatty acids are called "essential" because they cannot be made by the human body and must be consumed through the diet. The placement of the double bond in the carbon chain determines which class of fatty acids to which it belongs. The tail end of the carbon chain is referred to as the omega end and the placement of the double bond in relation to the omega end determines the type of fatty acid. Linoleic acid (LA) has its first double bond at the sixth carbon from the omega end, so it is a member of the omega-6 fatty acids:

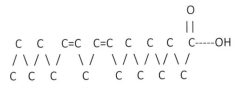

```
                                    O
                                    ||
    C   C   C=C  C=C  C   C   C   C-----OH
   / \ / \ /   \ /   \ / \ / \/ \ /
    C   C   C    C    C   C   C   C
```

Omega end   Alpha end

Linoleic acid (LA)

Other examples of omega-6 fatty acids include arachidonic acid (AA) and gamma linolenic acid (GLA) as illustrated below:

```
                    O
                    ||
    C = C   C = C    C   C-----OH
    /  \ /   \ /\ /
   /    C     C  C
  C
   \    C    C  C  C          Omega end
    \  /\   /\ /\ /
     C=C  C=C  C   C
```

Arachidonic Acid (AA)

```
    C=C   C   C
    /  \ / \ / \
   /    C   C  C-----OH
  /            ||
 C             O
  \
   \    C    C  C  C  C
    \  / \  / \ / \ / \ /    Omega end
     C=C  C=C   C   C   C
```

Gamma linolenic acid (GLA)

The omega-6 fatty acids are important in the human body since they are precursors to prostaglandins. They are the most common polyunsaturated fat found in foods. Gamma linolenic acid (GLA) is the most useful of these fatty acids in treating health problems since this omega-6 fatty acid can lead to the production of "good" eicosanoids. However, too much GLA can also lead to the production of "bad" eicosanoids such as arachidonic acid (AA) which leads to pain, swelling and inflammation. LA can be found in high amounts in seeds, corn and fish in warmer waters.

Alpha linolenic acid (LNA) is a member of the omega-3 fatty acids since the first double bond from the omega end is at the third carbon as illustrated below:

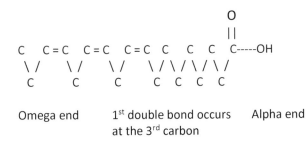

Omega end   1st double bond occurs   Alpha end
                   at the 3rd carbon

Alpha linolenic acid (Alpha linolenic acid)

Other examples of omega-3s include eicosapentenoic acid (EPA) and docosahexanoic acid (DHA):

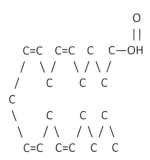

Eicosapentenoic acid (EPA)

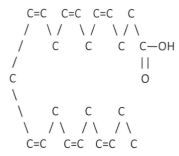

Docosahexanoic acid (DHA)

The omega-3 fatty acids are extremely important in the body. In addition to being precursors to prostaglandins, they help to keep cell membranes fluid and flexible which allows for effective exchange of nutrients in and out of the cell. Alpha linolenic acid, found primarily in plant foods, is converted in the body to EPA and DHA. Both EPA and DHA are critical for building neural tissue, but it appears that only DHA can stimulate the growth of nerve cells. DHA can actually cause the number of neuronal connections to increase. Omega-3s also promote vasodilation of blood vessels and have anti-inflammatory properties.

Several vitamins and minerals are necessary for the omega-3's to do their job and to help convert these fatty acids to prostaglandins. These include vitamins A, B, C, E and the minerals calcium, selenium, copper, zinc and manganese. The B vitamins help to boost the action of omega-3 fatty acids, and vitamin B6 is pivotal in helping to make prostaglandins; however, taking large doses of vitamin B with omega-3s should be avoided as this may greatly increase the effectiveness of this vitamin. Vitamin E helps to protect the EFAs from oxidation; calcium helps to stabilize nerve conduction; and selenium guards the fats in cell membranes.

Omega-3s should never be used to deep fry foods because the oil is destroyed resulting in the production of toxic substances.

Because these fatty acids are unsaturated, they will oxidize and turn rancid easily. Because of hydrogenation, the effectiveness of fatty acids has been destroyed which has led to a drastic reduction in these vital fats in the modern-day diet. In fact, Lipski (2000) states "Nearly half of our caloric intake comes from nutritionally depleted foods."

The National Institute of Health recommends the following daily intake of essential fatty acids:

EPA/DHA	650 mg.
LNA	2.22 g.
LA	4.44 g.

Rudin and Felix state that omega-3 fatty acids have decreased 80 percent in the past 100 years while omega-6 consumption has dramatically increased. This imbalance of omega-3 to omega-6 fatty acids lead to unbalanced levels of prostaglandins which can cause health problems. Our prehistoric ancestors were getting about a 1:1 ratio of omega-6 to omega-3 in their food; however, that ratio has changed in recent times. Today's diet has a ratio of 10:1 or even as high at 30:1 omega-6 to omega-3. As you can see, the modern diet supports the production of "bad" eicosanoids because of the large amounts of omega-6 fatty acids that are in our diet. In addition, trans-fatty acids can also cause a deficiency of omega-3 fatty acids.

Food processing has played a huge role in this imbalance of omega-6 to omega-3 fatty acids. In addition to the recognized problems with trans-fats, essential nutrients are being removed during food processing. For example, according to Lipski (2000), "Whole wheat contains twenty-two vitamins and minerals that are removed to make white flour. After the bran and germ are removed from the whole wheat kernel, so too are 98 percent of pyridoxine (vitamin B6), 91 percent of manganese, 84 percent of magnesium and 87 percent of fiber." She also reports that an average person eats 14 pounds of additives per year.

A study by B. Deutch done at Aarhus University in Denmark and published in the European Journal of Clinical Nutrition in 1995 looked at the level of menstrual pain associated with a low intake of omega-3 fatty acids. The researchers concluded that "results were highly significant and mutually consistent and supported the hypothesis that a higher intake of marine n-3 [omega-3] fatty acids correlates with milder menstrual symptoms" (Abstract). Another study by Harel, Biro, Kottenhahn and Rosenthal (1996) also showed a decrease in menstrual pain with dietary supplementation of omega-3 fatty acids. They concluded "dietary supplementation with omega-3 fatty acids has a beneficial effect on symptoms of dysmenorrhea in adolescents" (Abstract).

Several studies have shown a decrease in endometriosis symptoms when omega-3 fatty acid consumption is increased. A study done by Covens, Christopher and Casper (1988) demonstrated this finding in rabbits. The authors showed that "dietary supplementation with fish oil, containing the n-3 polyunsaturated fatty acids EPA and DHA, can decrease intraperitoneal PGE2 and PGF2-alpha production and retard endometriotic implant growth in this animal model of endometriosis"(Abstract). In another study done by Gazvani, Smith, Haggarty, Fowler and Templeton (2001), the researchers concluded "omega-3 PUFA [polyunsaturated fatty acids] may have a suppressive effect on the in vitro survival of endometrial cells, and omega-3 PUFA may be useful in the management of endometriosis by reducing the inflammatory response and modulating cytokine function" (Abstract). A third study done by Tomio et al. (2013) at the University of Tokyo also showed a protective effect of omega-3 fatty acids in the development of endometriosis. The results of their study showed "that both endogenous and exogenous EPA-derived PUFAs protect against the development of endometriosis through their anti-inflammatory effects and, in particular, the 12/15-LOX pathway products of EPA may be key mediators to suppress endometriosis" (Abstract).

However, a literature review by Parazzini, Vigano, Candiani and Fedele (2013) stated that the results of these studies could not be consistently replicated. The authors state, "a protective effect on endometriosis risk has been suggested for vegetable consumption and omega-3 polyunsaturated fatty acid intakes, whereas a negative impact has been reported for red meat consumption and trans fats and coffee intakes, but these findings could not be consistently replicated" (Abstract).

Another study by Missmer, Chavarro, Malspeis, Bertrone-Johnson and Hornstein (2010) looked at dietary fat consumption and not just the intake of omega-3s. Interestingly, they found that "although total fat consumption was not associated with endometriosis risk, those women in the highest fifth of long-chain omega-3 fatty acid consumption were 22% less likely to be diagnosed with endometriosis compared with those with the lowest fifth of intake...those in the highest quintile of trans-unsaturated fat intake were 48% more likely to be diagnosed with endometriosis..." (Abstract). They concluded that this "provides another disease association that supports efforts to remove trans-fat from hydrogenated oils from the food supply" (Abstract).

A study done by Khanaki et al. (2012) performed as a Ph.D. thesis at Tabriz University of Medical Sciences in Iran showed specifically the EPA to AA ratio may be useful in determining the degree of endometriosis present. They concluded "the components and the types of the fatty acids in serum total phospholipids seem not to be a marker for endometriosis, but the EPA/AA ratio is a relevant factor to indicate severity of illness" (Abstract).

Overall, these studies show that there is more than likely a beneficial effect to adding omega-3 fatty acids to the diet of women with adenomyosis. I personally found them to be highly effective in dealing with adenomyosis.

The following foods contain excellent sources of omega-3 fatty acids:

Anchovies
Canola oil
Flaxseed
Herring
Mackerel
Olive oil
Wild pacific salmon
Sardines
Soybean oil
Tuna
Walnuts

Flaxseed or Fish Oil?

There is some disagreement over whether flaxseed (linseed) oil or fish oil is better when trying to consume more omega-3s LNA inhibits the delta 6-desaturase enzyme, and therefore the conversion of LNA to EPA and DHA is limited. However, according to Ingeborg et al. (1990), a study done in Germany determined that "a diet of linseed [flaxseed] oil (30 ml. daily) for four weeks raised the content of LNA by 200 percent, the level of EPA by 150 percent and the level of DHA by 70 percent. The human body seems capable of transforming linolenic acid into EPA. This change coincided with a significantly reduced production of platelet thromboxanes (clotting agents)."

In addition to high levels of omega-3 fatty acids, flaxseed contains the highest known source of lignans in any food. Lignans been shown to inhibit enzymes involved in estrogen production and are known to occupy estrogen receptors which block the activation of endogenous estrogen. In addition, studies have shown high levels of estrogen in the urine of those that eat flaxseed daily (Brooks et al., 2004). In fact, the researchers state "supplementation with flaxseed modifies urinary estrogen metabolite excretion to a greater extent than does supplementation with an equal amount of soy" (Abstract). The reason for this is thought to be from the high content of lignans and fiber in flaxseed which help to transport bad estrogen out of the body.

As far as fish oil, some people don't like to take it because of the fishy aftertaste. In addition, there is also some concern about possible toxins in fish oil. If you want to take fish oil instead of flaxseed, look for high-quality supplements. They may be more expensive, but you won't have the fishy aftertaste and the risk of contamination by toxic substances is lower.

Although food processing has helped society in terms of convenience and has resulted in a reduction of food borne illness due to microbial contamination, it has set off a new health dilemma. As previously stated, trans-fats produced through food processing have led to a dramatic rise in the amounts of omega-6 fatty acids consumed while the available omega-3 fatty acids in foods have rapidly declined. According to Andrew Weil (2000, pg. 88), "if the diet is top heavy in omega-6 fatty acids, those will compete for a necessary enzyme, blocking the synthesis of DHA." Not only are omega-3 fatty acids vital to reduce inflammation, but there also appears to be a link between a lack of these essential fatty acids and estrogen dominance. For these reasons, women with adenomyosis should include an omega-3 supplement to their daily routine and increase their consumption of omega-3 rich foods.

Chapter 20 - What Supplements Help? What Supplements Should be Avoided?

"The World Health Organization notes that of 119 plant-derived pharmaceutical medicines, about 74 percent were used in modern medicine in ways that correlated directly with their traditional uses as plant medicines by native cultures."

-Burton Goldberg

The following list of supplements are those that may help with the symptoms of adenomyosis. Please also refer to Chapter 18 for more information on phytoestrogens as some of these supplements fall into that category.

1. **Anise (Pimpinella anisum)**
    Common names: Aniseed
    Native region: Central and Southern Europe, Egypt, Cyprus, Syria and Russia
    Actions: Expectorant, insecticide, stimulant, aphrodisiac
    Cautions: Interacts with birth control pills, estrogen drugs and tamoxifen.

    This herb has historically been used to treat menstrual pain, ease childbirth, increase milk flow and increase sex drive. It also eases gas, colic and indigestion. WebMD (2016) reports anise is possibly effective for menstrual discomfort. However, WebMD (2016) also states anise has estrogen-like activity and is not recommended in women with hormone-sensitive conditions.

2. **B vitamins** – see Chapter 17.

3. **Black Cohosh (Cimifuga racemose)**
    Common names: Squawroot, Black snakeroot, Bugbane, Rattleroot
    Native region: Eastern United States and Canada
    Actions: Diaphoretic, diuretic, antispasmodic, antidepressant, sedative, anti-inflammatory

Cautions: Overdose may cause severe headaches, nausea, dizziness and vomiting. Avoid use during pregnancy, while nursing or in cases of breast cancer or liver disorders. This herb may interfere with birth control pills and hormone replacement therapy. If stomach upset occurs when taking this herb, try taking it with meals.

A member of the buttercup family, this herb has been used extensively by the North American Indians for snakebites and nerve pain. It has a long history of use for premenstrual syndrome, dysmenorrhea and amenorrhea. It has also been used during pregnancy and childbirth. It appears to regulate uterine contractions during childbirth and helps to ease menstrual cramping. The active constituent cimicifugan has antispasmodic and sedative properties, but these actions are only found in the fresh root, not in the dried form of the herb. The salicylates in black cohosh are anti-inflammatory; however, this substance may irritate the gastrointestinal tract. Von Zepelin (2002) report women who took Remifemin tablets (which contain black cohosh extracts) for six months showed no changes in LH, FSH, prolactin or estradiol levels. Liu, Burdette, and Xu (2001) showed black cohosh had no activity in estrogen receptor binding in S30 (breast cancer) and Ishikawa (endometrial) cells. Zava et al. (1998) report black cohosh has little estrogenic bioactivity and Seidl and Stewart (1998, Table 2) state there is "no evidence of estrogenic effect in study of uterine growth in immature mice...". Since black cohosh seems to help with menstrual discomfort but does not appear to increase estrogen levels, this herb may be quite useful in the treatment of adenomyosis.

For best results, use this herb along with dong quai.

4. Blessed Thistle (Cnicus benedictus)

Common names: St. Benedict thistle, holy thistle, spotted thistle
Native region: Asia and Mediterranean regions
Actions: Diuretic, astringent, emetic, antibacterial
Cautions: Excessive use can cause vomiting.

Blessed thistle was used in the Middle Ages to treat the Black Plague. It is very bitter and doesn't smell good, so it is commonly used along with other herbs. This herb is known to stimulate the liver, and it has been used to treat painful menstruation.

5. Cascara Sagrada (Rhamnus purshiana)
Common names: California buckthorn, sacred bark, chittim bark
Native region: Western North America
Actions: Laxative, astringent
Cautions: The fresh bark causes nausea and severe cramps. The United States Pharmacopeia (USP) requires the bark to be at least a year old before use. Overuse can cause nausea, vomiting and abdominal pain/cramping and is contraindicated in cases of Crohn's disease or ulcerative colitis. In addition, this herb is contraindicated in pregnancy or while nursing. Cascara has been known to interact with digoxin. Use with caution if taking thiazide diuretics or corticosteroids.

This bitter and astringent herb was first used by the Indians and became popular in the Pacific Northwest in the 1800s. The anthraquinone glycosides in the bark stimulate peristalsis in the colon which makes it good for chronic constipation and hemorrhoids. Cascara sagrada is also known for its tonic effects on the liver and gastrointestinal tract as it increases the secretion of bile. This herb also helps in cases of enlarged liver.

6. **Chia** – In addition to its high fiber content, chia contains high amounts of omega-3 fatty acids, vitamins and minerals. Also, this wonderful food has a very high antioxidant activity level, so it is very beneficial to the liver. In fact, studies have shown significant liver health benefits in rats. Chia has also been known to aid in weight loss.

7. **Damiana (Turnera diffusa)**
    Common names: Damiana
    Native region: Desert Northwest region of Mexico
    Actions: Laxative, diuretic, expectorant, hormone regulator, nervine
    Cautions: Overdose may cause insomnia and headaches. Damiana may interact with other herbs and supplements that alter progesterone levels. Excessive use may cause diarrhea. Avoid use if on diuretics or if diabetic as this herb may affect blood sugar levels.

    Known for its aphrodisiac properties, this herb may help with anxiety, depression, hot flashes, dysmenorrhea and night sweats. Damiana can also improve mood by helping to combat depression and anxiety. It may inhibit aromatase which is needed to convert androgens to estrogen. A 1998 study found that this herb had anti-estrogenic activity and, according to Zava et al. (1998), this herb is one of the six highest progesterone-binding herbs. It has also been noted that this herb may contain compounds similar to progesterone, so it may be useful in cases of adenomyosis.

8. **Dandelion root (Taraxacum officinale)**
    Common names: Wild endive, cankerwort, lion's tooth, pee-in-the-bed, fairy clock, blow ball, puff ball
    Native region: Western Europe, Mediterranean
    Actions: Laxative, diuretic, tonic, antispasmodic, anti-inflammatory

Cautions: Avoid if allergic to chamomile, ragweed or yarrow. Should be avoided in those with liver or gallbladder problems. May interact with other diuretics, lithium, ciprofloxacin and antacids.

Dandelion root is a powerful diuretic which could be quite helpful if you suffer from severe bloating due to adenomyosis. The bitter flavonoids in dandelion root appear to be responsible for its diuretic effect. An additional benefit is that while the action of the herb is a diuretic, it doesn't cause the body to lose large quantities of potassium, an unwanted side effect of diuretic drugs such as Lasix®. According to Zhi et al. (2007), this herb may be useful "for the clinical treatment of reproductive hormone-related disturbances" (Abstract). Dandelion also detoxifies the liver which helps to effectively eliminate estrogen. The active constituent taraxacin is known to stimulate the liver and gallbladder, and It has been used to treat cirrhosis, jaundice, hepatitis and gallbladder disease. This herb can alter the concentrations of certain antibiotics.

9. **Diindolylmethane (DIM)** – DIM, also known as diindolylmethane, is formed in the body by substances found in cruciferous vegetables. It may act like an estrogen and may increase the levels of good estrogen (Lam, 2015b). Although there is insufficient evidence of its effectiveness, this substance may help prevent breast or uterine cancer and may help reduce the symptoms of PMS. DIM has been used in cases of estrogen dominance; however, the research for this use is lacking. May interact with many different medications including but not limited to Flexeril®, theophylline, Inderal®, Talwin® and Haldol®. Consult a physician before use if taking a prescription medication.

10. Dong Quai (Angelica sinensis)

Common names: Dang gui, tang kuei
Native region: China
Actions: Diuretic, uterine stimulant, emmenagogue, adaptogen
Cautions: Dong quai interacts with blood thinners such as heparin and warfarin. Sensitivity to sunlight is increased if taken with St. John's Wort. Avoid use during pregnancy or if on hormone replacement therapy.

This wonderful herb has been used extensively in China as a tonic for women, and they claim that it increases blood flow to the female reproductive organs. It is an adaptogen which basically means that it brings everything in the body into balance. Zava et al. (1998) report that this herb did not inhibit the production of alkaline phosphatase which means it does not block the activity of progesterone. In addition, this group notes that this herb has very little estrogenic activity. This herb may suppress estradiol synthesis since saliva levels in women who take this herb are very low.

According to Mark Pederson in his book, *Nutritional Herbology*, "In one study using direct measurement of the myometrium, administration of dong quai enabled the contractions of the uterus to be more orderly. This may be the mechanism underlying its effectiveness in treating dysmenorrhea." This herb may be an effective supplement to try in cases of adenomyosis.

For best results, use this herb along with black cohosh.

11. **Evening primrose oil** – This type of oil is a natural source of gamma linolenic acid (GLA), a type of omega-6 fatty acid. GLA is a precursor to a type of prostaglandin. There are some reports evening primrose oil can affect estrogen levels, but no carefully conducted clinical trial has been able to confirm these reports. Interestingly, the University of Maryland Medical Center Complementary

and Alternative Medicine Guide (2016) states this supplement may help women with endometriosis.

Cautions: Evening primrose oil interacts with anticoagulant and antiplatelet drugs such as aspirin, ibuprofen, naproxen, heparin, warfarin, Plavix® and Voltaren®. It is also known to interact with anesthesia and phenothiazines. Those with epilepsy should avoid evening primrose oil.

12. False unicorn (Chamaelirium luteum)
Common names: Helonias, blazing star, fairy wand, devil's bit
Native region: Eastern North America
Actions: Tonic, astringent, diuretic
Cautions: Excessive intake can cause vomiting.

Native American women have used false unicorn to help prevent miscarriage, and it has also been used to balance hormone levels due to the actions of saponins. This herb has also been used in cases of infertility, menstrual problems and digestive issues. It has the ability to expel intestinal parasites. False unicorn is endangered, and it should only be used under the supervision of qualified health practitioners.

13. Fennel (Foeniculum vulagare)
Common names: Wild fennel, sweet fennel, Florence fennel
Native region: Italy
Actions: Carminative, antimicrobial, antispasmodic, diuretic
Cautions: Has been known to interact with ciprofloxacin. Avoid use during pregnancy.

A popular seasoning for fish, fennel is known to stimulate the secretion of digestive fluids. The antispasmodic action of this herb on smooth muscle probably comes from its flavonoid content. Fennel contains anethole, photoanethole and dianethole. All three of these substances are believed to have estrogenic properties. Fennel is known to increase milk secretion, increase sex drive, and it may impact hormone levels. However, not enough is known about the activity of this herb to be able to label it as beneficial or detrimental to women with adenomyosis.

14. Ginseng (Panax ginseng)

Common names: Panax, sang, five finger root, ren shen, Chinese ginseng
Native region: Korea and Northeast China
Actions: Adaptogen, aphrodisiac, stimulant, estrogenic
Cautions: Those with high blood pressure should avoid use of this herb. Interacts with caffeine, MAOIs, lithium, insulin and warfarin.

The root of this herb is used, and it contains high amounts of phytoestrogens. It increases a person's ability to handle stress and improves energy levels. In addition, ginseng is known to stimulate both the immune system and liver enzymes, and it may correct abnormal functions of the thyroid and adrenal glands.

Although ginseng has been reported to help with PMS and infertility, it may have an estrogenic effect due to the similarity of its active ingredient, ginsenoside, to estrogen (Seidl & Stewart, 1998). Also, there is a reported case of postmenopausal bleeding in a woman who applied a ginseng cream vaginally (Seidl & Stewart, 1998). Women with adenomyosis should only use ginseng under the supervision of a professional.

15. Goldenseal (Hydrastis canadensis)

Common names: Yellow root, orange root, turmeric root, eye root, Indian turmeric, Indian plant, eye balm

Native region: Eastern half of the United States
Actions: Antibiotic, astringent, vasoconstrictor, tonic, antiseptic, antibacterial, antiviral, sedative
Cautions: Do not use during pregnancy or in cases of kidney disease. Has been known to interact with doxycycline and tetracycline.

Goldenseal stimulates the liver and is helpful in detoxification. It also improves the appetite by stimulating bile production. Its vasoconstricting effects help to control menstrual bleeding. The active constituents hydrastine and berberine have sedative properties.

Although goldenseal has these wonderful effects, Zava et al. (1998) report that this herb blocked enzyme production by progesterone, and they labeled goldenseal as an anti-progestin. This herb should be used with caution or not at all in women with adenomyosis.

16. **Grape Seed Extract** – Discovered in 1951 by the French scientist Dr. Jacques Masquelier, this amazing supplement has been shown to be a potent aromatase inhibitor. The ability of this supplement to inhibit aromatase may be very beneficial to women who suffer from estrogen dominance. In a study by Kijma, Phung, Hur, Kwok, and Chen (2006), grape seed extract was shown to be a possible treatment in cases of hormone-dependent breast cancer. Grape leaves, especially the leaves of the red grape, have been shown to have astringent qualities, and this might be beneficial in treating heavy menstrual bleeding. In addition, the proanthocyanidins in grape seed extract are powerful antioxidants which can help keep the liver healthy. Although the data is insufficient, grape seed extract may also help in cases of premenstrual syndrome. This supplement can interfere with blood thinners, NSAIDS

and heart medications. Avoid use in bleeding disorders and for at least two weeks prior to having surgery.

17. Hops (Humulus lupulus)
Common names: Hops
Native region: Europe and North America
Actions: Calmative, nervine, sedative, hypnotic, diuretic, antispasmodic, antibacterial, expectorant, anti-inflammatory
Cautions: Do not use in cases of depression. Do not use with other sedatives.

The active constituents in hops, humulone and lupulone, have a very bitter taste but are anti-inflammatory. Hops stimulates the production of digestive fluids and has been shown to relax smooth muscle. It also helps to promote more restful sleep.

However, Zava et al. (1998) report that hops has estrogenic effects, and this herb showed significantly higher growth of breast cancer cells when compared to a control. Additionally, females that harvest hops have been known to develop amenorrhea. Therefore, it is probably best to avoid this herb in cases of adenomyosis.

18. Lemon Balm (Melissa officinalis)
Common names: Bee balm, sweet balm, balm, garden balm, cure-all, dropsy plant, melissa
Native region: Southern Europe, West Asia and North Africa
Actions: Antispasmodic, antihistamine, diaphoretic, antiviral
Cautions: Known to interact with thyroid hormones. Interacts with pentobarbital. Avoid use in cases of low thyroid, pregnancy and glaucoma.

Lemon balm has been used to treat nervousness, insomnia and depression. In addition, this herb helps to reduce menstrual cramps. The active constituent citronellal has sedative properties. It improves digestion, relaxes muscle spasms and has been used to treat indigestion and other digestive issues.

19. Licorice (Glycyrrhiza glabra)

Common names: Sweetwood, sweetwort, sweet licorice
Native region: Mediterranean region and Southwest Asia
Actions: Sweetener, aphrodisiac, expectorant, laxative, antibacterial, antispasmodic, estrogenic, emmenagogue, antifungal, anti-inflammatory
Cautions: Licorice increases sodium retention and potassium loss; therefore, it should not be used in those with cardiac or kidney issues. This herb interacts with a whole host of medications such as aspirin, ibuprofen, naproxen, digoxin, oral and topical corticosteroids, loop diuretics and interferon. Consult a professional before use.

Licorice is the most commonly used of all herbs in Chinese herbal medicine. Its active constituent glycyrrhizin is fifty times sweeter than sugar. It has been used as a uterine tonic and in cases of infertility.

Licorice is known to have hormonal activity. According to Mabey (1988), "In the body, glycyrrhizin yields glycyrhetinic acid, which has a similar structure to the hormones of the adrenal cortex. This may explain why licorice demonstrates potent anti-inflammatory and anti-arthritis effects similar to cortisone."

This herb is controversial for use in estrogen dominance in my opinion. Before I go any farther, I want to clarify that many licorice products in the United States contain anise which gives these products the licorice flavor, but they do not contain the actual licorice herb. In this section, I am discussing the actual licorice herb. First, according to Paul Bergner (2001) glycyrrhiza, a component of licorice, can increase progesterone levels in the form of 17-hydroxy-progesterone which is great news for those women suffering from estrogen dominance. In addition, other research has shown that a combination of licorice and peony may reduce prolactin levels. However, licorice may have some estrogenic activity as well, and WebMD.com (2016) recommends that it not be used in hormone-sensitive conditions. Also, according to Zava et al. (1998), this herb is one of the six highest estrogen-receptor binding herbs. This group also notes cell growth in breast cancer cell lines showed significantly higher growth when compared to the control cell line, and they list this herb as an anti-progestin since it blocked the induction of alkaline phosphatase. So, what do you do? It depends. If you have a family history of breast cancer or other hormonal cancers, it is probably best to avoid this herb. Since licorice does have both progesterone and estrogen activity, it might be worth a try in women without a history of hormone-related cancers. It's up to the reader.

Note: According to Lee and Hopkins (2004), "Many licorice tinctures come deglycyrrhinized, thus eliminating [the concern of sodium retention and high blood pressure], but also possibly eliminating many of the therapeutic effects they might have in balancing hormones."

20. Marshmallow (Althea officinalis)
Common names: Sweetweed, wymote
Native region: Europe, Central Russia, West Asia and North Africa

Actions: Expectorant, diuretic, antibacterial, anti-inflammatory

Cautions: Do not take any oral drug at the same time as marshmallow. May cause an increase in mucous production.

This herb is different from the confectionary that is found in grocery stores today. This is an herb that has mucilaginous and expectorant properties that soothe inflamed and irritated tissues, particularly those in the digestive tract. Marshmallow is also known to reduce inflammation.

21. **Magnesium** – see Chapter 17.

22. **Melatonin** – This hormone is produced in the pineal gland in the brain and is important in modulating our circadian rhythms. It is also a free radical scavenger. It helps with the proper functioning of the immune system and plays and important role in the regulation of sex hormones. Recent studies have shown this hormone may reduce binding to estrogen receptors while it increases binding to progesterone receptors. A study by Rato et al. (1999) showed melatonin interfered with the activation of an estrogen receptor by estradiol. Abd-Allah, El-Sayed, Abdel-Wahab, and Hamada (2003) showed a 59 percent reduction of estrogen receptor binding in rats that were treated with melatonin. In addition, this same group showed an increase in progesterone receptor binding of 53 percent in these same rats. Melatonin interacts with sedatives, birth control pills, diabetic medications, caffeine and antiplatelet/anticoagulant drugs such as aspirin, ibuprofen, naproxen, Plavix® and Voltaren®.

23. **Milk Thistle (Silybum marianum)**
Common names: Holy thistle, St. Mary's thistle
Native region: Middle East

Actions: Antioxidant, tonic, diuretic, prevents liver damage

Cautions: Milk thistle may interfere with the effectiveness of birth control pills. It may also cause vomiting and diarrhea if consumed in excess. This herb may interfere with acetaminophen, general anesthesia, nitrous oxide, chemotherapy drugs, methotrexate, Lovastatin®, Pravastatin®, haloperidol, metronidazole, paclitaxel, cisplatin, tacrine and clofibrate.

Milk thistle refers to the milky sap that comes from the leaves and stems of this plant. This amazing herb has been known for thousands of years to protect and nourish the liver. It has bitter, tonic and diuretic activity. Silymarin is the active constituent of the plant, and this substance protects the liver from damage by toxins in several ways. First, it is a strong antioxidant, and it has been shown to be more effective than both vitamin C and vitamin E. Second, it helps to prevent the depletion of glutathione which is needed for the proper functioning of the liver. Lastly, this herb inhibits the production of enzymes that lead to the development of free radicals and leukotrienes, and it also stimulates the regeneration of liver cells.

Silymarin has been repeatedly shown to be beneficial in treating cirrhosis, fatty liver, jaundice and hepatitis. Since estrogen is processed in the liver, it is vital to keep the liver healthy, so the addition of this herb to the diet of adenomyosis patients is an excellent idea.

24. Motherwort (Leonurus cardiaca)

Common names: Lion's ear, lion's tail, Roman motherwort

Native region: Europe, South and Central Russia

Actions: Sedative, diuretic, antibacterial, antifungal, nerve tonic
Cautions: Do not take during pregnancy.

Motherwort has been used to regulate the menstrual cycle and to treat infertility. This herb has been used for amenorrhea. Tao et al. (2009) state Chinese motherwort ethanol extract may inhibit the proliferation of breast cancer cells. This group also states motherwort "markedly suppressed the development of uterine adenomyosis and mammary cancers in mice" (Abstract). In addition, this herb decreases muscle spasms and helps to soothe the nervous system. However, Zava et al. (1998) report that this herb has possible estrogenic effects, and growth of breast cancer cells were significantly higher as compared to control. Due to the conflicting data on this herb, it may not be a good idea to use it to treat adenomyosis at the current time.

25. Mullein (Verbascum thapsus)
Common names: Verbascum flowers, flannel flower, moth mullein, velvet leaf, lady's foxglove, Aaron's rod, donkey's ears, great mullein, Jacob's staff
Native region: Western Europe
Actions: Astringent, expectorant, diuretic, sedative, analgesic, antiseptic
Cautions: May increase mucous production.

The mucilage content of this bitter herb is soothing to inflamed and irritated tissues. It has been used primarily for respiratory disorders. It also has diuretic and expectorant properties.

26. N-acetyl-cysteine (NAC) – This supplement is an excellent antioxidant and chelator of heavy metals. It also aids in optimum liver function. NAC is derived from

the amino acid cysteine which contains a good amount of sulfur.

27. **Nutmeg** – Zava et al. (1998) report that this herb blocked enzyme induction by progesterone and have labeled it as an anti-progestin. Therefore, women with adenomyosis should use nutmeg sparingly.

28. **Omega-3 fatty acids** – see Chapter 19.

29. **Oregano** – According to Zava et al. (1998), oregano is one of the six highest progesterone-binding herbs. In addition, the volatile oils in oregano help to detoxify the liver. Since this herb may lower blood sugar levels, use with caution in cases of diabetes. Oregano may also interact with lithium.

30. **Pennyroyal (Mentha pulegium)**
Common names: Pudding grass, lurk-in-the-ditch, mosquito plant, squaw balm, squaw mint, tickweed
Native region: Europe, North Africa, Middle East
Actions: Diaphoretic, astringent
Cautions: The oil is toxic. Should not be used in cases of pregnancy, kidney disease or liver disease. Should never be given to infants.

Pennyroyal stimulates the uterus and promotes menstruation. This bitter herb should only be used under supervision and should probably be avoided in women with adenomyosis. Zava et al. (1998) report that this herb blocked enzyme induction by progesterone and have labeled it as an anti-progestin.

31. **Psyllium fiber (Plantago psyllium)**
Common names: Fiber, fleaseed
Native region: Mediterranean region
Actions: Bulk laxative, astringent

Cautions: Do not use in cases of bowel obstruction or intestinal narrowing. Interacts with lithium, levothyroxine and insulin.

This fiber supplement is found quite commonly in drug stores and is touted for its ability to help with constipation. The outer husk of psyllium seeds is the active part, and the astringent and cooling properties can be attributed to its active constituent, mucilage. When psyllium seeds are soaked in water, their size increases 8 to 14 times their original size. This increases bulk which stretches the intestinal tract and promotes peristalsis. The mucilage in psyllium is also known to absorb toxins in the digestive tract. Be sure to drink plenty of water when taking psyllium.

32. **Pycnogenol** – Use of 30 mg. of this supplement twice a day has been shown to significantly reduce pain in endometriosis patients. Pycnogenol can be found in chocolate, almonds, grape seeds, blueberries and cranberries.

33. **Quercetin** – This plant flavonoid is a strong aromatase inhibitor. A study done by van der Woude et al. (2005) showed that quercetin exerts phytoestrogen-like activity in the body. This group states "the results point at the relatively high capacity of quercetin to stimulate supposed 'beneficial' ER [estrogen receptor] beta responses as compared to the stimulation of ER [estrogen receptor] alpha, the receptor possibly involved in adverse cell proliferative effects" (Abstract). Quercetin is found in red wine, green tea, onions, berries and apples. It works best when taken with vitamin C. Excessive use can cause headaches and tingling in the arms and legs. Consultation with a physician is imperative if taking prescription medications as there are

many interactions. Some examples include cipro, cyclosporine, Zantac®, Tagamet® and Allegra®.

34. Red raspberry leaf (Rubus idaeus)

Common names: European red raspberry, American raspberry, wild red raspberry
Native region: England
Actions: Tonic, astringent, antispasmodic
Cautions: Red raspberry interacts with many medications including ephedrine, pseudoephedrine, theophylline, aminophylline, atropine, codeine, Cardec DM® and Lomotil®. Avoid use during pregnancy.

Used by the Chinese to strengthen the kidneys, red raspberry leaf's astringent properties are due to its tannin and fruit acid (citric and malic) content. This herb has been used as a female tonic as it is known to tone the uterine and pelvic muscles. Its constituent fragarine helps to balance out uterine peristalsis which may help to reduce dysmenorrhea. It also helps to reduce excessive menstrual bleeding. In addition, red raspberry is a rich source of manganese, magnesium, calcium and iron. This herb would be an excellent addition to the diet of women with adenomyosis.

35. Red Clover (Trifolium pretense)

Common names: Trefoil, cow grass, wild clover, cleaver grass
Native region: Europe, Western Asia, Northwest Africa
Actions: Diuretic, antispasmodic, estrogenic, relaxant, expectorant
Cautions: This herb is known to interact with a whole host of medications including but not limited to estrogens, birth control pills, tamoxifen and blood thinners such as heparin and warfarin. Avoid use during pregnancy.

The high content of isoflavones in red clover are converted into phytoestrogens in the body. The evidence of its usefulness is scarce, and there is a warning to avoid this herb in cases of hormone-sensitive conditions. The leaves are rich in estrogenic substances, and this herb is known to promote menstrual bleeding. In fact, according to Zava et al. (1998), red clover is one of the six highest estrogen-receptor binding herbs in their study. In addition, this group also notes that the potency of red clover is similar to estradiol. Therefore, it is probably wise to avoid this herb in cases of adenomyosis.

36. **Rosemary** – According to the Cleveland Clinic (2016), rosemary may lower estrogen levels. This herb also has anti-inflammatory properties, and its volatile oils aid in liver detoxification. Since rosemary may be toxic to embryos (Cleveland Clinic, 2016), avoid use during pregnancy or if trying to become pregnant. This herb may interact with lithium.

37. **Royal Jelly** – This nutritious supplement is made from bees. The major constituent is water (67%), but it also contains many nutrients such as protein, sugars, fatty acids, minerals, enzymes, vitamin B5, vitamin B6 and a small amount of vitamin C. It has been used for PMS, insomnia, menopause and liver disease. Royal Jelly has also been reported to decrease inflammation and nourish the endocrine system. According to Hiroyuki et al. (2012), this supplement appears to have no effect on the conversion of aromatase in humans. Caffeic acid phenethyl ester (CAPE) is a substance that is found in bee propolis. Jung et al. studied CAPE in 2010 and found that it had binding affinity to ERβ (estrogen receptor β). Also, CAPE did not increase the growth of MCF-7 estrogen receptor-positive breast cancer cells, and it did not increase uterine weight. There is a risk of allergic reactions with this supplement. There have been reports

of asthma, hives and even anaphylaxis, so use this supplement with caution especially if you have a history of allergies. Avoid use if taking warfarin or if pregnant.

38. **SAMe** – Also known as s-adenosyl methionine, this substance is made in the body as a result of a reaction between methionine and ATP. Methionine must be supplied through the diet as the body cannot make it. SAMe is an excellent source of sulfur and helps to convert estradiol (E2) into the less harmful estriol (E3). SAMe has been used for PMS and premenstrual dysphoric disorder (PMDD), a more severe form of PMS. It has also been used to help with depression and may even be useful in liver disease. SAMe has anti-inflammatory properties and has been used to relieve pain. An interesting study by Frezza, Tritapepe, Pozzato and Di Padova (1988) looked at the use of SAMe in women who had a history of liver disease called intrahepatic cholestasis of pregnancy (ICP). These women have an increased sensitivity to estrogen. They concluded "The data support the belief that SAMe acts as a physiological antidote against estrogen hepatobiliary toxicity in susceptible women" (Abstract). Do not use if you have bipolar disorder or Parkinson's disease. May interact with dextromethorphan, antidepressants (including MAOIs), St. John's Wort, levodopa, Demerol®, Talwin® and Ultram®. Since so little evidence is available for this supplement, it is highly advised to consult a physician before use. It is also advised to take folic acid and vitamin B6 with this supplement as excessive intake of methionine alone has been linked to stroke and heart disease.

39. Sarsaparilla (Smilax officinalis)
Common names: Quay, quill, spignet, Honduran sarsaparilla
Native region: Central and South America

Actions: Antiseptic, anti-inflammatory
Cautions: This herb is known to interact with digoxin and bismuth subsalicylate.

Used as a flavoring for root beer, this herb is a blood purifier that works mainly in the large intestine. The steroidal saponins in this herb bind endotoxins and helps to eliminate them through the bowel. Sarsaparilla herb stimulates the adrenal gland and may be useful in balancing hormones. It has also been used in liver disorders.

40. Senna (Cassia senna)

Common names: Locust plant, wild senna, purging cassia, American senna
Native region: Africa and Arabian Peninsula
Actions: Laxative
Cautions: Overuse can cause nausea, vomiting and abdominal pain/cramping. Contraindicated for use in cases of digestive disorders such as Crohn's disease, ulcerative colitis or intestinal obstruction. Its use is also contraindicated in pregnancy and in nursing mothers. Interacts with digoxin, thiazide diuretics and corticosteroids.

This herb is a laxative and is used to treat constipation. The anthraquinones promote intestinal peristalsis which usually results in a bowel movement in six to eight hours of consuming senna. It can be harsh, and it is recommended to be used sparingly. Due to its harshness, it is sometimes given with a carminative herb such as ginger to help with abdominal cramping. Using it alone will cause severe cramping. Senna is believed to be more habit-forming than cascara sagrada.

41. Slippery Elm (Ulmus fulva)

Common names: Red elm, moose elm, Indian elm

Native region: United States and Canada
Actions: Astringent, expectorant, anti-inflammatory
Cautions: Possible allergic reactions. Discontinue use in case of rash, itching or trouble breathing.

This mucilaginous herb is soothing and helps to draw out toxins from the body. It is useful in a whole host of digestive issues. The inner bark has been used as a survival food, and it is also an excellent food for those who are sick. The mucilage in this herb is soothing and anti-inflammatory. In addition, slippery elm contains a good amount of fiber.

42. Soy

Common names: Tempeh, miso, tofu, soymilk
Native region: Eastern Asia
Actions: Estrogenic
Cautions: Interacts with thyroid medications, MAOI antidepressants, antibiotics, warfarin, tamoxifen estrogen drugs and hormone replacement therapy.

Soy is a very complicated topic when it comes to its effect on hormone levels. There are many misconceptions about this food. The interest in soy and hormone levels came about because Asian women had a much lower risk of breast cancer than women in the United States. In fact, women in East Asia eat about ten times more soy than women in the U.S., but their hormone-positive breast cancer rates are far lower. This topic was discussed on the Dr. Oz show (2015) as they tried to clear up some misconceptions. They stated that soy can reduce breast cancer risk if eaten on a regular basis. However, in women who already have breast cancer, this benefit is questionable, so soy consumption is cautioned. They also state that the best types of soy are edamame, tofu and fermented soy products. Kurzer et al. (Abstract, 2002) states "soy and isoflavone consumption does not seem to affect endometrium in pre-menopausal women…". Additionally, Barret (2006) states that soy inhibits aromatase and inhibits angiogenesis. She also states a study showing that genistein, a component of soy, may inhibit the growth of breast cancer cells.

In contrast, some animal studies have shown consumption of large amounts of soy reduced fertility and triggered premature puberty. A study done by Jefferson, Padilla-Banks and Newbold (2007) report mice that were give genistein neonatally showed altered ovarian function and reduced fertility. Zava et al. (1998) lists soy as one of the six most potent estrogen-binding products. However, they also note that genistein suppresses estradiol synthesis. It is advised that women with adenomyosis who are considering adding soy to their diet do so with caution and after consultation with a natural health care practitioner.

43. **Thyme** – Zava et al. (1998) reports this herb as one of the six highest estrogen-receptor binding herbs, but it is also listed as one of the six highest progesterone-binding herbs. The volatile oils in thyme aid in liver detoxification. WebMD (2016) says to avoid use of this herb in hormone-sensitive conditions such as endometriosis. Since thyme is one of the six highest progesterone binding herbs, it might be safe to use this herb in small amounts in women with adenomyosis. Interacts with anticoagulants and antiplatelet drugs such as aspirin, ibuprofen, naproxen, Plavix® and Voltaren®.

44. Turmeric (Curcuma longa)
Common names: Indian saffron, hairdra
Native region: India
Actions: Astringent, antibacterial, anti-inflammatory
Cautions: Turmeric may interact with antiplatelet or anticoagulant drugs such as aspirin, ibuprofen,

naproxen, Plavix® and Voltaren®. Use with caution in gallbladder disease, diabetes, gastroesophageal reflux disease (GERD) and bleeding disorders.

Turmeric is an excellent anti-inflammatory supplement. Its active ingredient, curcumin, has been shown to be a powerful antioxidant. WebMD (2016) reports even though curcumin may act like estrogen in the body, studies have shown it may reduce the action of estrogen in hormone-sensitive cancer cells. However, evidence is limited, so its use is cautioned.

45. Vitex (Vitex agnus castus)

Common names: Chasteberry, chaste tree, monk's pepper, agnus castus, hemp tree
Native region: Mediterranean, Central Asia
Actions: Astringent, relaxant
Cautions: This herb should not be used in those with Parkinson's disease, those who have schizophrenia, women who are undergoing in vitro fertilization, women who are nursing or women who are pregnant. May interact with birth control pills, estrogens, medication for Parkinson's disease, antipsychotic medications and Reglan®. Avoid if using bromocriptine.

This herb is also known as "the woman's herb" and is known for its hormone-balancing effects. It influences the pituitary gland to produce luteinizing hormone which, in turn, signals the ovaries to produce progesterone. Vitex may also lower prolactin levels. It has been used to treat fibrocystic disease, abnormal menstrual bleeding, PMS, PMDD, polycystic ovarian syndrome (PCOS), uterine fibroids, miscarriage, low progesterone levels, menopausal symptoms and infertility. In a 1988 study, researchers investigated the effects of this herb in women with luteal phase defect (low progesterone levels in the last half of the menstrual cycle). Forty-five women with this defect took vitex once a day for three months, and progesterone levels returned to normal in 25 of the women (WholeHealthMD.com, 2005). This group also states this herb may help to relieve endometriosis pain. According to Seidl and Stewart (1998), this herb was found to be effective in cases of hyperprolactinemia. In addition, vitex appears to be comparable in effectiveness to Prozac in the treatment of PMDD. This herb may help women with adenomyosis.

46. Vitamin E – see Chapter 17.

47. Zinc – see Chapter 17.

Section V

Chapter 21 - How Does Stress Play a Role in Adenomyosis?

"If your cortisol is chronically high, you'll have overall resistance to your hormones. It's essential to address the stress factor if you want to achieve hormone balance."

- Dr. David Zava

In Chapter 3, I discussed how cortisol levels influence the levels of other hormones. As previously discussed, the health of the adrenal glands is of utmost importance in maintaining proper cortisol levels. In this chapter, I will further describe how stress affects hormonal balance.

The adrenal glands are two small glands that sit on top of the kidneys and are heavily involved in how our bodies react to stressors. Stressors are any events which sets off the "fight or flight" response. Examples include marriage, divorce, moving, death, and daily stressors such as traffic, illness or job stress. Each adrenal gland is divided into two parts – the adrenal medulla and the adrenal cortex. The function of the adrenal medulla is to give the body a quick response to stressors. It releases epinephrine which increases heart rate and breathing. In addition, it increases the amount of sugar pumped into the bloodstream which gives the body a quick burst of energy. In contrast, the function of the adrenal cortex is to respond to chronic stress. This part of the gland produces mineralocorticoids and androgens which are substances that help the body to respond to longer-term stressors. The glucocorticoids are cortisol and hydrocortisone. They regulate blood sugar levels, muscle function and inflammation. The mineralocorticoids include aldosterone, and progesterone is a precursor to aldosterone, thus the importance of progesterone in adrenal gland function. These substances regulate mineral balance.

When a person is under stress, impulses from the sympathetic nervous system (which originate in the hypothalamus) raise the concentration of glucose in the blood. This in turn increases breathing and heart rate. Stress also increases the release of epinephrine from the adrenal medulla. While all this is going on, the hypothalamus stimulates the anterior pituitary to release ACTH which, in turn, increases cortisol levels.

Sources of Stress

- Job loss
- Financial problems
- Change of job
- Moving
- Environmental toxins
- Not enough sleep
- Poor diet
- Illness
- Divorce
- Deadlines at work or home
- A packed schedule without any "down time"

When too much cortisol is present, blood sugar levels fluctuate resulting in weight gain, especially in the abdomen. Since most people are stressed constantly these days, the cortisol levels often remain consistently high which can lead to a condition called adrenal fatigue.

Symptoms of Adrenal Fatigue

- Digestive issues
- Fatigue
- Allergies
- Premenstrual syndrome
- Low sex drive
- Hyperglycemia leading to insulin resistance
- High blood pressure
- Immune system dysfunction
- Mood swings, depression, anxiety, and feeling overwhelmed due to pressure
- Easy bruising
- Osteoporosis

Cortisol competes with progesterone receptors. This means that if cortisol levels are high, they will occupy progesterone receptor sites which will ultimately lead to low progesterone levels since progesterone will not be able to lock into the receptors and activate. To make matters even more complicated, if the level of E2 (estradiol) is low, this will lead to increased levels of cortisol which, in turn, will lower progesterone levels. I hope it is becoming increasingly clear that all hormone levels need to be at optimal levels for the entire system to work well.

Factors That Increase Cortisol Levels

- Infections
- Not enough sleep
- Exposure to toxins
- Birth control pills
- Inflammation and chronic pain

When too little cortisol is present, it results in fatigue and menstrual abnormalities. This fatigue can be manifested as a person having trouble getting out of bed in the morning. High mineralocorticoid levels lead to mineral imbalance, water retention and high blood pressure.

Balance of all these substances are vital to hormone balance. In fact, an imbalance of cortisol levels have been noted to appear as a thyroid problem. According to Zava in an interview with Dr. John Lee and Virginia Hopkins (2004), "A lot of people who have an imbalance in adrenal cortisol levels usually have thyroid-like symptoms but normal thyroid levels." So, if your thyroid levels are normal but you still have symptoms, it is worth it to look at the adrenal glands and cortisol levels.

As stated above, progesterone is a precursor to aldosterone. According to Zava in an interview with Lee and Hopkins (2004), "...progesterone plays an important role because it's the only natural hormone that actually competes with cortisol for glucocorticoid receptors. It can counter the stimulating effects of cortisol at night when you need to be sleeping."

Adrenaline is also known to interact with progesterone. High adrenaline levels can block progesterone receptors preventing progesterone from being used in the body.

Ways to Support Healthy Adrenal Glands

- Stress management
- Get enough sleep
- Supplement with vitamin B5 (pantothenic acid), vitamin C and licorice root

Ways to Reduce Stress Levels

1. Make sure you eat well. Include foods with high levels of B vitamins, vitamin C, magnesium and zinc, manganese and copper.
2. Meditation
3. Massage and/or reflexology
4. Take a hot bath
5. Read your favorite book
6. Take a break during the day – drink a cup of coffee or tea or take a short nap if possible
7. Listen to your favorite music while you work
8. Go for a walk – clear your mind and enjoy the sounds of nature
9. Take gentle exercise classes for stress reduction – yoga and tai chi are excellent choices
10. Get a full night of sleep. Researchers at the University of Chicago (Lee and Hopkins, 2006) showed that those who slept 6.5 hours a night had 50 percent more insulin resistance than those who slept 8 hours. In addition, other research showed an increase in inflammation in those who were short on sleep.
11. Prayer
12. Learn breathing exercises
13. Dancing
14. Counseling or talking to a friend
15. Avoid environmental toxins as much as possible.
16. Get a pet
17. Do some type of aerobic activity at least three times per week.

Chapter 22 - Why are Women with Adenomyosis so Emotional?

"You wake up every morning to fight the same demons that left you so tired the night before, and that, my love, is bravery."

– unknown

Well, I think we all now know why they are so emotional. The hormonal imbalances associated with adenomyosis clearly play a major role.

I want to share the emotional side of my own story. I have noticed that many doctors and nurses tend to focus predominately on the physical symptoms of both adenomyosis and endometriosis without addressing the emotional aspects of this disorder.

In the first few years of dealing with adenomyosis, I became incredibly frustrated at not getting a definitive diagnosis. I was told, after all the clinical testing and exams, that I had irritable bowel syndrome. I was told this was a diagnosis of exclusion because everything else they tested for came back negative. This made me angry and frustrated because I felt they were basically telling me "all testing is negative, so we're going to slap this diagnosis on the problem since we really have no idea what is wrong with you."

Some of my co-workers knew what I had gone through, and instead of comforting me through one of the most difficult journeys of my life, they chose to judge me. Since the doctors couldn't figure out what was wrong, they automatically jumped to the conclusion that I was making it all up. Whenever I called out sick because of the severe pain, the next day at work, I saw several of them huddled together and talking and when they would see me, they would stop talking and walk away. I knew what was being said because friends of mine told me. It's awful to not have a diagnosis, but to have other people look at you and think that you're the problem...well, that's just the icing on the cake.

331

I became so depressed that on some days, I could barely get out of bed. I hated going to work. On some days, I don't know which was worse – the pain from adenomyosis, not having a definite diagnosis or having to tolerate the whispering behind my back at work. I eventually quit my job because the stress level from all of this was just too much for me.

Several years later, as I was recovering from yet another night of excruciating abdominal pain, nausea, vomiting, diarrhea and severe bloating, I told my mom that I was so desperate for a definite diagnosis that I would be happy if they told me I had cancer. At least I would have an answer.

I began to have panic attacks. I was afraid that all the pain and gastrointestinal issues would flare up suddenly when I was in traffic or on a plane or anywhere where I couldn't quickly get home or to a bathroom. On several occasions, I cried driving to and from work when I was stuck in traffic. At home, I was depressed, moody and impatient because I had a significant other that did not understand what I was going through, and I felt like he didn't want to understand. I can't tell you the number of times I heard, "well, other women handle it...why can't you?" I felt incredibly alone. I recall one night when I had one of my worst attacks. I heard him get up (it was about 3 a.m.), and I thought to myself, "Good, he knows I am not in bed, so surely he will check on me and take me to the hospital." Well, he didn't. Instead he went back to bed. I was in so much pain and so weak that I could not make it to the bedroom to ask for help. I was completely and utterly alone. I cried most of that night not only because I was in so much pain but also because I felt like I had no one. It is a horrible place to be.

In doing research for my books, I have learned that other women have felt the same depression, frustration, and incredible loneliness that I went through during my ordeal. In fact, there have been cases of women with these disorders that have felt so helpless that they have committed suicide. This should never, ever happen! But I will be honest – I completely understand the desperation that these women felt.

The Endometriosis Foundation of America has started a wonderful program called EMPOWR. They educate teenagers on endometriosis, and they include boys in the program. Padma Lakshmi, one of the founders of the Endometriosis Foundation of America, explained in a video about how important it is for boys to understand this disorder as well as girls. It is so important for the male population to be educated on both adenomyosis and endometriosis in case their girlfriend and/or wife has one of these disorders so that they will not contribute to the suffering of their girlfriend/wife by dismissing her symptoms. I encourage all who read this book to get involved with the EMPOWR program through this wonderful organization.

Obviously, it is incredibly important to address the physical aspects of adenomyosis. However, we must all remember that the emotional aspects are just as important. I believe that any good doctor or nurse should address both and not neglect the emotional side. It is incredibly important that these women have a safe place to go to vent their frustration and to find emotional support while dealing with this disorder. I have started an online support group through Adenomyosis Fighters where these women can vent as long as they are respectful to other members. That is my only rule for the group. I feel that by adding on a bunch of rules prevents the women from being open and honest, and I deeply understand the need to be able to be open honest since I went through it myself. My online support group can be found at https://www.facebook.com/groups/adenofighters/

Conclusion

"It is not easy to talk about a condition once dismissed as 'the career women's disease'. But women will continue to suffer until we realize the cost of ignoring it"

— Hilary Mantel

In a study performed by Taran et al. (2010), the authors concluded that "a better understanding of this disease is required to improve diagnosis and management" (Abstract, conclusion section).

One of the main issues is the lack of attention that this disorder has received. Owalbi and Strickler (1977) state "the common association of adenomyosis with more obvious pelvic disease has diminished its significance as a cause of gynaecologic symptoms. Adenomyosis is the addendum to textbook chapters on ectopic endometrium; it is the forgotten process and a neglected diagnosis" (as cited in Taran, 2013, Clinical Phenotype section, para. 2). Therefore, it is so important to raise awareness of this uterine disorder, not only in the medical field but also in the general public. When I tell people that I had adenomyosis for seventeen years, most of the time they give me a blank stare. But when I mention that it is like endometriosis, they recognize that term. Adenomyosis needs to be as recognizable a term as endometriosis.

One of the biggest problems in researching this disorder has to do with diagnostic criteria. According to Meredith, Sanchez-Ramos and Kaunitz (2009), it was very difficult to perform a meta-analysis on adenomyosis studies since different diagnostic criteria were used in each study. The group states "each study used different definitions of adenomyosis and included studies performed with different ultrasound transducers" (Comments section, para. 5). Accurate information cannot be obtained when the criteria are not consistent. The same group also discussed the actual ultrasound images and the criteria that were used in the meta-analysis saying "most studies included the findings of myometrial heterogeneity or a globular uterus as criteria, while others included the finding of myometrial cysts. Which criterion was most specific for adenomyosis varied between studies" (Comments section, para. 5). With different criteria being used in these studies, we are not able to get an accurate picture of adenomyosis. It is imperative that researchers come up with more stringent criteria to get a clearer picture of the disorder.

Another important issue regarding research has to do with the lack of high-quality studies. According to Guo (2012), one of the main reasons for the lack of reliable knowledge on adenomyosis is the failure of investigators to develop well-controlled studies. Guo states "less than desirable methodological quality of mouse efficacy studies of adenomyosis...could have contributed to the lack of progress in developing noel treatments for adenomyosis" (Methodological Qualities of Published Mouse Efficacy Studies section, para. 2). In addition, Guo (2012) points out that in May 2012, there were 389 publications on PubMed for adenomyosis as compared to 18,593 for endometriosis, Taran et al. (2013, Abstract, para. 1) states "...despite the clinical importance of adenomyosis, there is little evidence on which to base treatment decisions." The group concluded in their report that "prospective randomized and controlled studies with larger cohort, validated and disease-specific symptoms questionnaires, noninvasive diagnostic modalities as well as new surgical and interventional alternatives to hysterectomy are required to better understand adenomyosis and to avoid hysterectomy" (Conclusions section, para. 3). No wonder the physicians and ultrasound technologists are unable to diagnose this disorder accurately!

During my struggle with adenomyosis, the medications that were prescribed were of very little use to me. I suffered from severe abdominal pain each month, and I was desperate for something to take the edge off the pain. According to Guo (2012), adenomyosis is a "gynecological disorder with a poorly understood pathogenesis" and "more efficacious drugs with better side effect and cost profiles are sorely needed" (Abstract).

Progestins and GnRH agonists are of limited use. According to Guo (2012, Introduction section, para. 2), "progestogenic agents are not very effective, and GnRH agonists...use is restricted by short duration." It has been reported that adenomyosis does not effectively respond to danazol. Clearly, the women who suffer from adenomyosis need more effective ways to manage the pain each month. The current options give minimal relief at best.

Currently the only way to effectively "cure" adenomyosis is through hysterectomy. Many women opt for this even though they are years away from menopause because they can't take the monthly pain any longer. In addition, many of these women never have children due to the fertility issues involved. (Add info here on the new excision treatments and MRgFUS).

Another very important reason to determine better treatment options for adenomyosis is the high cost of health care for those who suffer from this disorder. As of 2013, the cost of hysterectomies in the United States were estimated to be 2.1 billion annually (Taran et al., 2013). According to an article published in The Guardian in 2015 by Jessica Glenza, the cost for healthcare the year after a woman is diagnosed with endometriosis was $13,199, and over a ten-year period, the healthcare cost was $26,305 higher than a woman who did not have endometriosis.

Insufficient funding for research is also a major concern. According to Glenza (2015), endometriosis funding received $7 million in 2014 from the National Institutes of Health (NIH). That number went down from 2011 when the funding was double that amount. In addition, Glenza (2015, para. 6) points out that in 2014, "for each person believed to have diabetes in the United States, the NIH spends $35.66 annually. For each woman with endometriosis, the NIH spends $0.92." Those figures are for endometriosis, not adenomyosis! Clearly adenomyosis is a significantly neglected, even ignored, uterine disorder.

Campo et al. (2012) state there is a "renewed interest by the scientific community on an otherwise neglected condition, creating a flurry of research activities leading also to improved knowledge of the relationship between adenomyosis and endometriosis" (Introduction section, para. 7). This is a very encouraging statement, and I hope that this "renewed interest" persists in the coming years. We desperately need more research, better treatment options and a consensus on the diagnostic criteria for adenomyosis.

Current Adenomyosis and Endometriosis Studies

The following clinical studies are recruiting participants. Please see https://clinicaltrials.gov for more information.

1. **Levonorgestrel-releasing Intrauterine System versus a Low-dose Combined Oral Contraceptive for Management of Adenomyosis Uteri**

   Location: Ain Shams University-Maternity Hospital, Cairo, Egypt

2. **High-intensity Focused Ultrasound in Treatment of Uterine Adenomyosis**

   Location: Queen Mary Hospital, Hong Kong, China

   Adenomyosis and Ulipristal Acetate

   Location AP-HP, Bicetre Hospital, Le Kremlin, Bicetre, France

3. **A Prospective Study of Diagnostic Accuracy of Ultrasound**

   Texas Tech University Health Science Center, El Paso, TX

4. **Development and Validation of EHP-30 (Hong Kong Chinese Version) for Patients with Endomeriosis and Adenomyosis**

   Location: The Chinese University of Hong Kong, Hong Kong, China

5. **The Association Between Adenomyosis/Uterine Myoma and Lower Urinary Tract Symptoms**

   Location: Far-Eastern Memorial Hospital, Banqiao, New Taipei, Taiwan

6. **Cooperative Adenomyosis Network**

   Location: Peking Union Medical College Hospital, Beijing, China

7. **Treatment of Benign Uterine Disorders Using High Intensity Focused Ultrasound (MR-HIFU)**

   Location: Turku University Hospital, Turku, Finland

The following studies are new but not yet recruiting. Keep an eye on these studies if you want to participate in them.

1. Effect of Ulipristal Acetate on Bleeding Patterns and Dysmenorrhea in Women with Adenomyosis

   Location: Vanderbilt University Medical Center, Nashville, TN

2. Comparison of Estrogen-progestin Therapy in Continuous Regimen Versus Combination Estrogen-progestin Therapy in Continuous Regimen Plus Levonorgestrel-releasing Intrauterine System (LNG-IUS)

   Location: University of Cagliari, Sardinia, Italy

The following studies have recently been completed, and we anxiously await the results:

1. **Histopathological Diagnosis of Adenomyosis**

Location: Kasr el aini Hospital, Cairo, Egypt

2. **Levonorgestrel-releasing Intrauterine System for the Treatment of Symptomatic Adenomyosis**

   Location: Peking Union Medical College Hospital (get location)

3. **Norwegian Adenomyosis Study I**

   Location: Oslo University Hospital, Oslo, Norway

4. **Vaginal Bromocriptine for Treatment of Adenomyosis**

   Location: Mayo Clinic, Rochester, MN, USA

5. **Aromatase Inhibitors or GnRH-a for Uterine Adenomyosis**

   Location: Mansoura University Hospitals, Mansoura, Dakahlia, Egypt

6. **Effectiveness of IV Acetaminophen and IV Ibuprofen in Reducing Post Procedural Pain in the UFE Procedure.**

   Location: UCLA Medical Center, Los Angeles, CA and Santa Monica/UCLA Medical Center and Orthopedic Hospital, Santa Monica, CA

7. **Use of Dexamethasone in Uterine Artery Embolization**

   Location: Department of Anesthesiology and Pain Medicine and Anesthesia and Pain Research Institute, Yonsei University College of Medicine, Seoul, South Korea

8. **Uterine Artery Embolization for Symptomatic Fibroids**

   Location: Health Sciences Centre, Winnipeg, Manitoba, Canada

9. **AMH Levels Change During Treatment with GnRH Agonist**

   Location: Chair of Obstetrics and Gynecology – University Division – UMG, Catanzaro, CZ, Italy

Recommended Physicians

USA

Dr. Andrew Cook

Honors: Internationally renowned endometriosis specialist, international lecturer, member of American Association of Gynecologic Laparoscopists (AAGL) and International Pelvic Pain Society, awarded "Special Excellence in Endoscopic Procedures, American Association of Gynecologic Laparoscopists"

Contact information: Vital Health Endometriosis Center, San Francisco, CA, USA, https://www.vitalhealth.com/#tophome, (408)358-2511

Dr. John Dulemba

Honors: Expert in the use of the daVinci robot, Medical advisor for the Endometriosis Association, Member of American Association of Gynecologic Laparoscopists, International Laparoscopy Association, Society of European Robotic Gynecologic Surgeons, Fellow of American College OB/Gyn, several publications

Contact information: The Women's Centre, Denton, TX, U.S.A., www.womenscentre.net, (940)387-6248

Dr. Charles Koh

Honors: Endometriosis excision specialist, double boarded in U.S.A. and England, Co-director, Milwaukee Institute of Minimally Invasive Surgery, Associate Clinical

Professor, Department of Obstetrics and Gynecology, Medical School of Wisconsin, voted World Class Doctor, Gynecological Laparoscopy, Milwaukee Magazine and Top Doctor, Infertility, Milwaukee Magazine

Contact information: Columbia St. Mary's Hospital, Milwaukee, WI, U.S.A. www.reproductivecenter.com, (414)289-9668

Dr. Thomas Lyons

Honors: Member of American Society of Reproductive Medicine, European Society for Gynaecologic Endoscopy, Australian/New Zealand Society of Gynaecological Endoscopy, on advisory board of American Association of Gynecologic Laparoscopists, on editorial board for *Gynecologic Endoscopy*, author and lecturer

Contact information: Center for Women's Care and Reproductive Surgery, Atlanta, GA, U.S.A. (770)352-0037

Dr. Cindy Mosbrucker

Honors: Endometriosis excision specialist, trained under internationally recognized Dr. David Redwine, specialist in urogynecology, member of the American Board of Obstetrics and Gynecology

Contact information: Pacific Endometriosis and Pelvic Surgery, Gig Harbor, WA, U.S.A., (253)313-5997

Dr. Camran Nezhat

Honors: Long history of performing some of the most difficult reproductive surgeries (please see his website), author of eight textbooks, teaches medical professionals from all over the world, received many awards from organizations such as the American College of OBGYN, American Society of Reproductive Medicine, Society Laparoendoscopy Surgeon and others.

Contact information: Center for Special Minimally Invasive and Robotic Surgery, Palo Alto, CA, www.nezhat.org, USA, (650)327-8778

Dr. Ceana Nezhat – Nezhat Medical Center

Honors: World-renowned gynecological surgeon, Adjunct Clinical Professor of Gynecology and Obstetrics at Emory University, Founder and Symposium Chair of the World Symposium on Endometriosis, co-author of several textbooks, widely sought-after lecturer

Contact information: Nezhat Medical Center in Atlanta, GA, USA. https://endometriosisspecialists.com, (404)255-8778 or (888)659-2311

Dr. Tamer Seckin

Honors: Internationally recognized leader in endometriosis care, lecturer, researcher, over 30 years of experience in excision surgery, Founder and Medical Director of the Endometriosis Foundation of America, awards include inclusion in Super Doctors, Best Doctors in America and many others. Recipient of the Ellis Island Medal of Honor. Member of numerous gynecological associations.

Contact Information: 872 5th Ave. New York, NY 10065, (212)988-1444

Dr. Ken Sinervo

Honors: Internationally recognized leader in endometriosis care, Rate MD's Top 10 Gynecologists in the World, Vitals.com Patient Choice Honor for five years in a row, Patient's Choice, awarded "Most Compassionate Physician", Chairman of Endometriosis and Reproductive Surgery Special Interest Group (SIG) of AAGL, member of numerous gynecological associations.

Contact Information: Center for Endometriosis Care, 6105 Peachtree Dunwoody Rd., Building B, Suite 230, Atlanta, GA 30328, (770)913-0001

England

Note: There are many endometriosis centres in the United Kingdom. I have listed a few below, but if you need a clinic that is not listed, please refer to the BSGE website at https://www.bsge.org.uk/centre for a comprehensive list of accredited endometriosis centres in England.

The Endometriosis Centre
University College London Hospitals
Elizabeth Garrett Anderson Wing
Clinic 3
Lower ground floor
235 Euston Road
London NW1 2BU
020 3447 9411/ 020 3447 9393
www.theendometriosiscentre.co.uk

Mr. Sanjay Vyas

Bristol Gynaecology
Spire Bristol Hospital (The Glen)
Redland Hill
Durdham Down
Bristol BS6 6UT
0117 980 4070
www.bristolgynaecology.com

Colchester Endometriosis Centre
Colchester Hospital University
Main Building
Turner Road
Colchester, Essex CO4 5JL
01206 747474
www.colchesterhospital.nhs.uk/obs_endometriosis.sht
ml

Dorset Endometriosis Centre
Poole Hospital NHS Foundation Trust
Longfleet Road
Poole BH15 2JB
https://www.poole.nhs.uk/a-z-
services/e/endometriosis-care.aspx

Australia

The Endometriosis Care Centres

Adelaide: **Dr. Susan Evans**
                    38 The Parade
                    Norwood SA 5067
                    08 8363 2811

Brisbane: **Dr. Graham Tronc**
                    Wesley Medical Centre
                    Suite 15, Level 1

40 Chasely Street
Auchenflower, QLD 4066
07 3870 5602
www.grahamtroncmedical.com.au

Gold Coast: John Flynn Medical Centre
Suite 3B
Island Drive
Tugun, QLD 4224
07 5598 0055

Melbourne: Suite 1, Harley Chambers
171 Victoria Parade
Fitzroy 3065
03 9415 6855

Perth: 10 Nicholson Street
Subiaco WA 6008
08 9382 8323

Sydney: **Dr. Geoffrey Reid**
Park House
Level 7
187-191 Macquarie Street
Sydney NSW 2000
1300 367 874

Dr. Jim Tsaltas
344 Victoria Parade
East Melbourne VIC 3002
(03)9416 1172
www.mivf.com.au

Dr. Jason Abbott
48-50 St. Paul's Street
Randwick, NSW 2031
02 9009 5255

www.alanahealthcare.com.au

Dr. Omar Adham
Canberra Endometriosis Centre
GPO Box 825
Canberra City ACT 2601
www.health.act.gov.au/our-services/women-youth-
and-children/gynaecology-and-womens-
health/canberra-endometriosis-centre

Centre for Advanced Reproductive Endosurgery

Care – St. Leonards
AMA House
Level 4, Suite 408
69 Christie Street, St. Leonards
Sydney NSW 2065

Care- Kogarah
St. George Private Hospital
Level 4, Suite 7
1 South Street
Kogarah NSW 2217

Canada

Dr. Liane Belland
#305-1010 1 Ave. NE Calgary
Calgary, AB, Canada
(403)266 3030

Dr. Terry Unger
200 Boudreau Road
St. Albert, AB, Canada
(780)459 1104

Dr. Christina Williams

University of British Columbia
Suite 930, 1125 Howe Street
Vancouver, BC Canada V6Z 2K8
(604)875-2445
www.obgyn.ubc.ca

Dr. Nicholas Leyland
1200 Main St.
W. Hamilton, ON L8N 3Z5
(905)521-2100
www.endometriosisclinic.ca

Iran

Avicenna Fertility Center
No. 97
Junction of Yakhchal St., Shari' ati St.
Tehran, Iran
+98 (21) 23 519
http://www.avicennaclinic.ir

Ireland

Altnagelvin Area Hospital Endometriosis Centre
6 Faughan View Park
Londonberry, Derry, United Kingdom BT47 2TA
028 7134 5171
http://www.westerntrust.hscni.net

Scotland

Professor Andrew Horne, Clinical Lead
EXPPECT Endometriosis Team at the University of
Edinburgh
Chalmers Health Centre

2A Chalmers Street
Edinburgh EH3 9ES
+44 (0) 131 242 6988
https://www.ed.ac.uk/centre-reproductive-
health/exppect-endometriosis/the-endometriosis-team

Switzerland

Dr. Jean-Marie Wenger
Roseraie Avenue 76A
1205 Geneva, Switzerland
+41 22 321 26 66
www.jmwenger.com

Singapore

A/Prof Bernard Chern
A/Prof Tang Heng Hao
Dr. Khoo Chong Kiat
Dr. Cynthia Kew
Dr. Anthony Siow
Dr. Jasmine Mohd
KK Endometriosis Centre
Gleneagles Medical Centre #05-04
6 Napier Road
Singapore 258499
(65)6479 9555
www.anthonysiow.com/

Africa

International Centre for Minimal Access Surgery
1st Floor Parklands MediPlaza
3rd Avenue, Parklands
P.O. Box 38291
Nairobi, Kenya 00623

+254-20-3749040/20
www.laparoscopyicmas.com

Dr. Sulaiman Heylen
209 Library Square
1 Wilderness Road
Claremont, 7708
Cape Town, South Africa
+27 21 674 2088
www.capefertility.co.za

Japan

Dr. Yutaka Osuga
The University of Tokyo Hospital
7-3-1 Hongo, Bunkyo-ku
Tokyo 113-8655 Japan
www.h.u-tokyo.ac.jp

Israel

The Chaim Sheba Medical Center at Tel Hashomer
52621 Ramat Gan
Israel
03 5303295
https://eng.sheba.co.il

Germany

Dr. Med. Garri Tchartchian
114129 Berlin
Kurstrasse II
030 809 88 431
https://meindoctor.com

Brazil

Dr. Mauricio Abrão
Ruã São Sebastião
550-Chacara Santo Antõnio
04708-001 São Paulo
(11)5180-3344
www.drmauricioabrao.com

Abbreviations

4-MBC – 4-methylbenzylidine camphor
β-HCH – β-hexachlorocyclohexane
AA – Arachidonic acid
ATP – Adenosine triphosphate
BCP – Birth control pill
BHA – Butylated hydroxy anisole
BPA – Bisphenol A
BPS – Bladder pain syndrome, AKA interstitial cystitis or bisphenol S
CA19-9 – Cancer antigen 19-9
CA125 – Cancer antigen 125
CAPE – Caffeic acid phenethyl ester
COX 2 – Cyclo-oxygenase 2
CSF – Cerebrospinal fluid
D&C – Dilation and curettage
DDT – Dichlorodiphenyltrichloroethane
DEHP – di(2-ethylhexyl) phthalate
DES – Diethylstilbestrol
DGLA – Dihomogamma linolenic acid
DHA – Docosahexanoic acid
DIM – Diindolylmethane
DNG - Dienogest
E1 – Estrone
E2 – Estradiol
E3 – Estriol
EA – Endocrine activity
EDC – Endocrine disruptor
EFA – Essential fatty acid or Endometriosis Foundation of America
EMI – Endometrial/myometrial interface (junctional zone)
EPA – Eicosapentenoic acid or Environmental Protection Agency
ERα – Estrogen receptor alpha
ERβ – Estrogen receptor beta
FSH – Follicle stimulating hormone

GLA – Gamma linolenic acid
GnRH – Gonadotropin-releasing hormone
hCG – Human chorionic gonadotropin
HETE – Hydroxyeicosatetraenoic acid
HLA – Human leukocyte antigen
HRT – Hormone replacement therapy
I3C – Indole-3-carbinol
IBS – Irritable bowel syndrome
IC – Interstitial cystitis
IL-6 – Interleukin-6
IUD – Intrauterine device
IV – Intravenous
IVF – In vitro fertilization
JZ – Junctional zone
LA – Linoleic acid
LH – Luteinizing hormone
LNA – Alpha-linolenic acid
LT – Leukotriene
LUNA – Laparoscopic uterosacral nerve ablation
Lx - Lipoxin
MAOI – Monoamine oxidase inhibitor
MMP-2 - Matrix metalloproteinase 2
MMP-9 – Matrix metalloproteinase 9
MRgFUS – Magnetic resonance-guided focused ultrasound
MRI – Magnetic resonance imaging
MRSA – Methicillin-resistant staphylococcus aureus
NAC – N-acetyl cysteine
NSAID – Non-steroidal anti-inflammatory drug
OCP – Organochlorine pesticide
Oxo-ETES - Oxoeicosanoids
PBB – Polybrominated biphenyl
PCB – Polychlorinated biphenyl
PCOS – Polycystic ovarian syndrome
PFD – Pelvic floor dysfunction
PG – Prostaglandin
PGE2 – Prostaglandin E2
PGF2 – Prostaglandin F2 alpha

PGI - Prostacyclin
PID – Pelvic inflammatory disease
PL - Prolactin
PMDD – Premenstrual dysphoric disorder
PSN – Presacral neurotomy
PUFA – Polyunsaturated fatty acid
RCT – Randomized controlled trial
Rv - Resolvin
SAMe – S-adenosyl methionine
SHBG – Sex-hormone binding globulin
SLS – Sodium lauryl sulfate
SPM – Specialized pro-resolving mediators
STIP1 – Stress-induced phosphoprotein 1
TIAR – Tissue injury and repair
TVS – Transvaginal sonogram
TX - Thromboxane
UAE – Uterine artery embolization
US – Ultrasound
USP – United States Pharmacopeia
VEGF – Vascular endothelial growth factor

Definitions

17-OH-pregnenolone – Formed by the hydroxylation of pregnenolone, this prohormone is converted into DHEA.

17-α-OH- progesterone – a hormone related to progesterone that is converted into other hormones in the body.

β-hexachlorocyclohexane (β-HCH) – a type of organochlorine pesticide.

Adaptogen – an herb that increases resistance to stress

Adenocarcinoma – cancer that arises from glandular tissue

Adenomyoma – abnormal mass of endometrial tissue found within the myometrium. An adenomyoma is usually benign and is associated with adenomyosis.

Adenosine trisphosphate (ATP) – a substance that is a part of energy transportation in cells as a part of the process of metabolism.

Adhesion – abnormal union of two separate tissues because of inflammation.

Adrenal fatigue – condition where the adrenals are not functioning at the optimum level. It is characterized by unrefreshing sleep and is usually caused by chronic stress or infection.

Adrenal gland – Two endocrine glands that sit on top of the kidney. They produce a variety of hormones.

Agonist – a chemical that stimulates action.

Aldosterone – the main mineralocorticoid that is produced by the adrenal cortex.

Alpha-linolenic acid (LNA) – a type of omega-3 fatty acid that can be converted into EPA and DHA in the body. It is an essential fatty acid which means it must be included in the diet.

Amenorrhea – absence of menstruation.

Analgesic – a substance that relieves pain.

Androgen – a hormone that regulates the development of male characteristics.

Androstenedione/androstenediol – steroid hormones that are intermediaries in the production of estrogen and testosterone.

Anemia – low levels of hemoglobin present in red blood cells. Since hemoglobin is involved in the transport of oxygen throughout the body, low levels can cause fatigue, dizziness, headache, shortness of breath, and cold intolerance. One cause of anemia is excessive blood loss from abnormally heavy menstruation.

Angiogenesis – the growth of new blood vessels in the human body.

Antihistamine – a substance that block the action of histamine. Antihistamines are useful in controlling allergies.

Anovulation – failure of the ovary to release an egg.

Antagonist – a substance that interferes with the action of another substance.

Antibacterial – chemical that kills bacteria.

Antifungal – chemical that kills fungi.

Anti-inflammatory – an herb that soothe inflamed tissues.

Antimicrobial – an herb that helps the body to destroy disease-causing microorganisms.

Antioxidant – a molecule that inhibits oxidation, thereby reducing free radical formation.

Antispasmodic – an herb that help to ease cramping.

Aphrodisiac – substance that increases sexual desire.

Apoptosis – programmed cell death necessary for the proper functioning of the human body.

Arachidonic acid (AA) – a type of omega-6 fatty acid that is a vasodilator and is heavily involved in the inflammatory process.

Aromatase – an enzyme that converts androgens to estrogen in the body.

Astringent – a substance that shrinks body tissues.

Benign – not cancerous.

Bioactivity – the effect of a substance on living tissue.

Bioidentical progesterone cream – a type of cream that contains progesterone that is identical to endogenous progesterone on a molecular level.

Biopsy – removal of a small piece of tissue from the body. It is then analyzed under a microscope to determine if an abnormality is present or not.

Calmative – a substance that has a sedative or calming effect.

Cancer antigen 19-9 (CA19-9) – tumor marker for pancreatic cancer.

Cancer antigen 125 (CA125) – marker that detects early stages of ovarian cancer.

Carcinogen – substance that causes cancer.

Carminative – a substance that expels gas.

Cervix – cylindrical-shaped tissue that separates the uterus from the vagina.

Chelator – a compound that can bind to a metal. Chelators are used to help eliminate metal toxins from the body.

Circadian rhythm – a 24-hour cycle of physical and mental changes that respond to light and dark.

Cirrhosis – damage to the liver that causes a reduction in its functional capabilities.

Cohort – a group of people in a study.

Corpus luteum – a small yellow body formed from an ovarian follicle after the egg has been released at ovulation. It secretes progesterone in order to support a pregnancy; however, if pregnancy does not occur, the corpus luteum will degenerate, and a new menstrual cycle will begin.

Cortisol – steroid hormone that is released from the adrenal glands in response to stress.

Cystic – related to or containing cysts.

Cytochrome P450 – hemoproteins that are involved in the metabolism of toxins in the body. Most of these hemoproteins are found in the liver.

Dehydroepiandrosterone (DHEA) – precursor to testosterone and estrogen.

Detoxification cleanse – process of using nutrients to help eliminate toxins from the body.

Diaphoretic – a substance that induces sweating.

Dienogest – a semi-synthetic progestin. It has been used to treat endometriosis under the name "Visanne".

Dihomogamma linolenic acid (DGLA) – a fatty acid that is involved in the production of anti-inflammatory eicosanoids.

Diuretic – a substance that encourages fluid loss from the body by increasing urine output.

Diverticulitis – infected or inflamed pouches (diverticula) on the wall of the colon Symptoms include gas, bloating, constipation, diarrhea, abdominal pain, loss of appetite, and nausea.

Docosahexanoic acid (DHA) – a type of omega-3 fatty acid that is found in cold water fatty fish.

Dysmenorrhea – painful menstrual bleeding.

Echotexture – characteristic pattern seen on radiology images.

Ectopic – occurring in an abnormal place; out of proper position.

Ectopic pregnancy – a pregnancy that occurs outside of the uterus, usually in the fallopian tube. This is a dangerous condition and should be promptly treated as it can cause internal bleeding and possible death.

Eicosanoid – a molecule that is made from omega-3 and omega-6 fatty acids. Prostaglandins, leukotrienes, thromboxanes and lipoxins are examples. They are heavily involved in the inflammatory process in the body.

Eicosapentenoic acid (EPA) – a type of omega-3 fatty acid that is found in cold water fatty fish.

Emetic – a substance that induces vomiting.

Emmenagogue – an herb that stimulates menstrual flow.

Endocrine disruptor – chemicals that cause hormonal imbalance by interfering with the proper functioning of the endocrine system.

Endogenous – substance made by the human body. Endogenous progesterone is that which is made by the body.

Endometrial carcinoma – uterine cancer that begins in the endometrium.

Endometrioma – a cyst that is formed on the ovaries due to displaced endometrial tissue. Also called a "chocolate cyst" because of its deep red/brown appearance, endometriomas are found in patients suffering from endometriosis.

Endometrium – the inner lining of the uterus that responds to hormonal stimulation.

Epithelium – closely packed cells that line the interior and exterior surfaces of the body. An example is the skin. It is one of the four major tissue types of the human body.

Essential fatty acid (EFA) – fats that can't be synthesized by the human body and must be included in the diet. LNA and LA are examples of essential fatty acids.

Estradiol (E2) – the most potent form of estrogen produced by the human body. It is the predominant form of estrogen during the reproductive years. The level of estradiol drops after menopause.

Estriol (E3) – a type of estrogen that is produced by the placenta and is abundant during pregnancy.

Estrogen – sex hormone responsible for the development and maintenance of female characteristics and reproduction. Plays a major role in the menstrual cycle.

Estrone (E1) – the least abundant type of estrogen. It is less potent than estradiol and is the major form of estrogen found in menopausal women. Estrone can be converted into estradiol.

Expectorant – a substance that enhances the expulsion of mucous.

Fallopian tube – the tube connecting the ovary to the uterus. The egg travels down this tube after being released from the ovarian follicle at ovulation.

Fibrocystic breast disease – non-cancerous cysts in the breast. The cysts can be solid (fibrosis) or fluid-filled, and their growth is stimulated by estrogen.

Fibroid – a benign tumor of the uterine smooth muscle. Also referred to as a leiomyoma, it can cause heavy periods, infertility and anemia.

Follicle-stimulating hormone (FSH) – hormone produced in the anterior pituitary gland that is responsible for the maturation of ovarian follicles.

Free radical – an atom with at least one unpaired electron. It is highly reactive and can damage cells.

Gamma linolenic acid (GLA) – a type of omega-6 fatty acid. It can be converted into AA in the body. A good source of GLA is evening primrose oil.

Gonadotropin – a hormone that stimulates the gonads. FSH and LH are examples of gonadotropins.

Hepatitis – inflammation of the liver.

Hepatobiliary – refers to the combination of the liver, gallbladder and bile ducts.

Herbicide – chemical used to kill unwanted plants.

HOX genes – genes that control the development of the basic structure of the body. Also called homeotic genes.

Hydroxyeicosatetraenoic acid (HETE) – A type of eicosanoid that sends white blood cells to the site of tissue injury

Hyperplastic – an increase in the number of normal cells in an organ or tissue. These cells may also be larger than normal.

Hyperprolactinemia – higher than normal levels of prolactin in a female's body. Can cause oligomenorrhea, amenorrhea and infertility.

Hypertrophic – excessive growth of an organ or tissue.

Hyperthyroidism – Overactivity of the thyroid gland resulting in increased metabolic activity and enlargement of the gland.

Hypnotic – a substance that induces deep sleep.

Hypothalamus – Region of the brain that is the main control center of the autonomic nervous system. It is also an endocrine gland that is involved in hormone production and secretion.

Hypothyroidism – an underactive thyroid. The gland doesn't produce enough thyroid hormone which leads to fatigue, weight gain, depression and constipation.

In vitro – tests conducted in an artificial environment outside of a living organism. The term is Latin for "within the glass".

In vivo – tests performed on living tissue. The term is Latin for "within the living".

Insecticide – a chemical used to kill insects.

Interleukin 6 (IL-6) – chemicals that are actively involved in the inflammatory process and act as pyrogens.

Irritable bowel syndrome (IBS) – disorder of the colon that can cause abdominal pain, cramping, bloating, constipation and/or diarrhea. IBS is a diagnosis of exclusion which means that the physician must rule out all other known causes of these symptoms before this diagnosis can be given. IBS is a functional disorder of the colon due to abnormal peristalsis, and it is not life-threatening. Adenomyosis and endometriosis are known to quite often be misdiagnosed as IBS.

Isoflavones – strong antioxidants that have estrogen-like activity in the body.

Laxative – a substance that loosens stools and promotes easier bowel movements.

Leiomyoma – see Fibroid.

Leukotriene – A lipid produced by white blood cells. Leukotrienes are produced in allergies and other inflammatory reactions.

Lignans – Found in plants, these substances are the main sources of phytoestrogens in the modern-day diet. Bacteria break down lignans in the intestinal tract to substances that have weak estrogen activity.

Linoleic acid (LA) – a type of omega-6 fatty acid that can be converted to GLA and AA in the body. This type of fatty acid is essential and must be included in the diet.

Lipoxin – eicosanoid that helps to reduce inflammation.

Luteal insufficiency – a condition where the uterine lining fails to grow properly each month. This is due to low progesterone levels or the failure of the uterine lining to respond properly to progesterone. This condition may cause fertility issues and is also referred to as "luteal phase defect".

Luteinizing hormone (LH) – a hormone produced in the anterior pituitary gland. A surge in LH occurs in the last half of the menstrual cycle and is responsible for ovulation and the development of the corpus luteum.

Macrophage – a type of large white blood cell that is involved in the destruction of foreign invaders such as bacteria and viruses.

Malignant – cancerous.

Menarche – the first menstrual cycle.

Menorrhagia – abnormally heavy menstrual bleeding.

Meta-analysis – an analysis that uses statistics to combine findings from two or more studies.

Metabolite – an intermediate substance produced during metabolism.

Microcyst – a cyst that can only be seen with a microscope.

Monoamine oxidase inhibitor (MAOI) – a type of antidepressant.

Mucilage – a viscous or gelatin-like substance.

Mucilaginous – a sticky substance that secretes mucilage.

Müllerian ducts – embryonic ducts that develop into fallopian tubes, uterus, cervix and vagina.

Mutation – a permanent change in a DNA sequence.

Myometrial ectopic pregnancy – a pregnancy that occurs within the uterine myometrium. This condition is rare, but when it does occur, it could cause uterine rupture.

Myometrium – The outer muscular layer of the uterus.

Neoplastic – abnormal growth of tissue that can be either malignant or benign.

Nervine – an herb that promotes the health of the nervous system.

Oligomenorrhea – infrequent or very light menstrual periods.

Ovarian cyst – a solid or fluid-filled sac on the surface or within the ovary. Most do not cause symptoms; however, if he cysts are large or have ruptured, they can cause pelvic pain, painful intercourse, nausea and vomiting.

Ovarian follicles – a spherical group of cells found in the ovary. They secrete hormones and hold oocytes which eventually develop into eggs.

Oxoeicosanoids (oxo-HETEs) – eicosanoids that send white blood cells to the site of tissue injury.

Oxytocin – a hormone that helps to regulate childbirth and breast-feeding. It is produced in the hypothalamus and stored in the posterior pituitary gland.

Pathogenesis – the mechanism of the development of a disease.

Pelvic inflammatory disease (PID) – an infection caused by bacteria that has made its way through the cervix and into the rest of the female reproductive tract. Symptoms include lower abdominal pain, abnormal vaginal discharge, nausea and vomiting. It is usually sexually transmitted.

Peristalsis – involuntary rhythmic contractions that move contents through a tubular organ such as the intestines.

Peritoneum – the membrane that lines the walls of the abdomen and protects the abdominal organs.

Pesticide – a chemical that kills any kind of pest. Herbicides and insecticides are two types of pesticides.

Pituitary gland – a pea-sized gland located at the base of the brain. It controls the functioning of endocrine glands and is involved in the production of several different hormones in the body. Also referred to as the "master gland".

Placenta – An organ that functions in pregnancy. It provides nourishment to the fetus.

Polycystic ovarian syndrome (PCOS) – an ovarian disorder in which many small cysts develop on the ovaries. This is due to a hormonal imbalance caused by excessive levels of androgens. Symptoms include excess body hair, weight gain, infertility and irregular periods.

Polyunsaturated fatty acid (PUFA) – a type of fat that has more than one unsaturated carbon bond. These fats are liquid at room temperature and solid when refrigerated. Examples include omega-3 and omega-6 fatty acids.

Pregnenolone – a 21-carbon steroid produced from cholesterol. It is a precursor to sex hormones.

Premenstrual dysphoric disorder (PMDD) – a severe form of premenstrual syndrome.

Proanthocyanidins – a type of flavonoid found in plants. They are antioxidants and are known to be beneficial in the treatment of cardiovascular disease, diabetes and cancer.

Progesterone – female sex hormone that plays a major role in the menstrual cycle.

Progestins – synthetic steroid hormones that bind to progesterone receptors and activate them.

Prolactin – a hormone that simulates the production of breast milk. The pituitary gland makes it.

Prospective trials – a study that follows a group over a set period of time.

Prostacyclin – a prostaglandin that inhibits platelet aggregation and functions as a vasodilator.

Prostaglandin – a type of lipid that controls the contraction and relaxation of smooth muscle, modulates inflammation and regulates blood flow. It is made from arachidonic acid, a type of omega-6 fatty acid.

Pyrogen – a substance that induces fevers.

Randomized controlled trials – studies where people are randomly placed in groups that receive different treatments. An example is a study of the usefulness/side effects of a medication. One group is a control group that will receive a placebo, and the other group is the experimental group that will receive the medication. Those involved in the study do not know who is receiving the placebo and who is receiving the actual medication. This is the most common type of scientific study performed since it minimizes bias.

Relaxant – a substance that causes relaxation.

Sedative – a substance that induces sleep.

Speculum – an instrument that looks like the "beak of a duck" and is used to spread open the walls of the vagina during a pelvic examination by a gynecologist.

Stimulant – an herb that invigorates the activity in the body.

Submucosal – connective tissue that lies beneath a mucous membrane

Subperitoneal – located beneath the peritoneum.

Surfactant – a substance that reduces the surface tension of a liquid allowing it to foam and penetrate solids.

T-cells – a type of white blood cell that is heavily involved in immune system function.

Tamoxifen – a medicine used in the treatment of breast cancer.

Testosterone – a male sex hormone. It is also present in small amounts in females.

Thromboxane – compounds that constrict blood vessels and cause blood to clot.

Thyroid – an endocrine gland that makes and stores hormones.

Tonic – an herb that nurtures the overall health of the body.

Trans-fatty acid- manufactured fatty acids that are dangerous to health. These fats are created through a process called hydrogenation.

Uterine hyperperistalsis – a condition where uterine contractions are more frequent than those seen in a normal uterus.

Uterine implantation – the adherence of a fertilized egg to the wall of the uterus.

Uterine polyp – mass that originates from the endometrium. It can be flat up against the uterine wall or may be pedunculated (on a stalk). Polyps can grow up to several centimeters and may be associated with heavy menstrual bleeding. Also referred to as an "endometrial polyp".

Vascularization – development of blood vessels through natural or surgical means.

Vasoconstrictor – a substance that causes blood vessels to contract which in turn stops bleeding.

Recommended Reading

What Your Doctor May Not Tell You About Menopause: The Breakthrough Book on Natural Hormone Balance by Dr. John Lee and Virginia Hopkins

Dr. John Lee's Hormone Balance Made Simple by Dr. John Lee and Virginia Hopkins

What You Must Know About Women's Hormones: Your Guide to Natural Hormone Treatments for PMS, Menopause, Osteoporosis, PCOS, and More by Pamela Wartian Smith, MD, MPH

Is It Me or My Hormones? By Marcelle Pick, MSN, OB/GYN NP

Recognizing and Treating Endometriosis: The Doctor Will See You Now by Dr. Tamer Seckin

Alternative Medicine by Burton Goldberg

Eating Well for Optimum Health by Andrew Weil, MD.

The Omega Rx Zone by Dr. Barry Sears

Prescription for Herbal Healing by Phyllis Balch, CNC

References

Adb-Allah, A.R.A., El-Sayed, E.S.M., Abdel-Wahab, M.H., & Hamada, F.M.A. (2003). Effect of melatonin on estrogen and progesterone receptors in relation to uterine contractions in rats. *Pharmacological Research. 47(4),* 349-54. doi: 10.1016/S1043-6618(03)00014-8

Agency for Toxic Substances & Disease Registry (2018). Public Health Statement for Aldrin/Dieldrin. Retrieved from www.atsdr.cdc.gov/phs/phs.asp?id=315&tid=56

Agency for Toxic Substances & Disease Registry (2018). Public Health Statement for Endosulfan. Retrieved from www.atsdr.cdc.gov/phs/phs.asp?id=607&tid=113

Agency for Toxic Substances & Disease Registry (2018). Public Health Statement for Hepatachlor and Hepatachlor Epoxide. Retrieved from www.atsdr.cdc.gov/phs/phs.asp?=743&tid=135

Agency for Toxic Substances & Disease Registry (2018). Public Health Statement for Methoxychlor. Retrieved from www.atsdr.cdc.gov/phs/phs.asp?id=776&tid=151

Agency for Toxic Substances & Disease Registry (2018). ToxFAQs for Dichlorobenzenes. Retrieved from www.atsdr.cdc.gov/toxfaqs/tf.asp?id=703&tid=126

Agency for Toxic Substances & Disease Registry (2018). ToxFAQs for Polybrominated Biphenyls. Retrieved from www.atsdr.cdc.gov/toxfaqs/tf.asp?id=528&tid=94

Albee, R. B. (2016). Adenomyosis: Is it really endometriosis? Center for Endometriosis Care. www.centerforendo.com/adenomyosis-is-it-really-endometriosis

Amazon.com (2018). Crystal Star Women's Vegetarian Capsules. Retrieved from https://www.amazon.com/Crystal-Star-Womens-Vegetarian-Capsules/dp/B00028LX88

Baccionttini, L., Falchetti, A., Pampaloni, B., Bartolini, E., Carossino, A.M. & Brandi, M.L. (2007). Phytoestrogens: Food or drug? *Clinical Cases in Mineral and Bone Metabolism, 4(2),* 123-130. Retrieved from http://www.ncbi.nlm.nih.gov/pmc/articles/PMC27812344

Badawy, A.M., Elnashar, A.M., & Mosbah, A.A. (2012). Aromatase inhibitors or gonadotropin-releasing hormone agonists for the management of uterine adenomyosis: a randomized controlled trial. *Acta Obstetricia Gynecologica Scandinavica, 91*, 489-495. doi: 10.1111/j.1600-0412.2012.01350.x

Barleans Organic Oils, LLC (2003). Natural healing with flax: Important help for diabetics. Retrieved from http://www.barleans.com/literature/flax/83-help-for-diabetics.html

Barrett, J.R. (2006). The science of soy: What do we really know? *Environmental Health Perspectives, 114(6)*, A352-A358. Retrieved from http://www.ncbi.nlm.nih.gov/pmc/articles/PMC1480510/

Barton-Schuster, D. (2015). Herbs and supplements with estrogen action Q&A. Message posted to http://natural-fertility-info/herbs-and-with-supplements-estrogen-action-qa.html

Bazot, M., Cortez, A., Darai, E., Rouger, J., Chopier, J., Antoine, J.M., & Uzan, S. (2001). Ultrasonography compared with magnetic resonance imaging for the diagnosis of adenomyosis: Correlation with histopathology. *Human Reproduction, 16(11)*, 2427-33. Retrieved from http://ncbi.nlm.nih.gov/pubmed/1167953

Beck, V., Unterrieder, E., Krenn, L., Kubelka, W. & Jungbauer, A. (2003). Comparison of hormonal activity (estrogen, androgen and progestin) of standardized plant extracts for large scale use in hormone replacement therapy. *Journal of Steroid Biochemistry and Molecular Biology, 84(2-3)*, 259-68. Retrieved from http://www.ncbi.nlm.nih.gov/pubmed/12711012

Behera, M.A. & Gest, T.R. (2011). Uterus anatomy. In Medscape. Retrieved from http://emedicine.medscape.com/article/1949215-overview#al

Benagiano, G.P., Brosens, I.A., Carrara, S., & Filippi, V. (2010). Adenomyosis. In *The Global Library of Women's Medicine*. ISSN: 1756-2228. doi: 10.3843/GLOWM.10460

Benagiano, G., Brosens, I., & Carrara, S. (2009). Adenomyosis: New knowledge is generating new treatment strategies. *Women's Health, 5(3)*, 297-311. Retrieved from http://www.medscape.com/viewarticle/703820_5

Bergeron, C., Amant, F., & Ferenczy, A. (2006). Pathology and physiopathology of adenomyosis. *Best Practices and Research Clinical Obstetrics and Gynaecology, (20)4*, 511-21. Retrieved from https://www.ncbi.nlm.nih.gov/pubmed/16563870

Bergner, P. (2001). Glycyrrhiza: Licorice root and testosterone. *Medical Herbalism, 11(3),* 11-12. Retrieved from http://www.medherb.com/Materia_Medica/Glycyrrhiza_-_Licorice_root_and_testosterone.htm

Beta-catenin. Retrieved April 13, 2015 from Wikipedia: http://en.wikipedia.org/wiki/Beta-catenin

Bioscience Technology (2013). Closing in on Cause of Adenomyosis. Retrieved from http://www.biosciencetechnology.com/news/2013/10/closing-cause-adenomyosis

Biggerstaff, E.D. & Foster, S. (1994). Laparoscopic presacral neurectomy for treatment of midline pelvic pain. *The Journal of Minimally Invasive Gynecology, 2(1),* 31-35. doi: 10.1016/S1074-3804(05)80828-X

Board on the Health of Select Populations, Institute of Medicine, Washington, DC. (2014). Committee to Review the Health Effects in Vietnam Veterans of Exposure to Herbicides. National Academies Press (US).

Boue, S.M., Wiese, T.E., Nehls, S., Burow, M.E., Elliott, S., Carter-Wientjes, C.H.,...Cleveland, T.E. (2003). Evaluation of the estrogenic effects of legume extracts containing phytoestrogens. *Journal of Agricultural and Food Chemistry, 51(8),* 2193-9. Retrieved from http://www.ncbi.nlm.nih.gov/pubmed/12670155

Bown, D. (2001). Encyclopedia of Herbs. U.S.: DK Publishing, Inc.

Bratby, M.J, & Walker, M.J. (2009). Uterine artery embolization for symptomatic adenomyosis – mid-term results. *European Journal of Radiology. 70(1),* 128-132. doi: 10.1016/j.ejrad.2007.12.009

Brinker, F. (2001). Herb Contraindications & Drug Interactions. U.S.: Eclectic Medical Publications

Bromley, B., Shipp, T.D., & Benacerraf, B. (2000). Adenomyosis: Sonographic findings and diagnostic accuracy. *Journal of Ultrasound in Medicine, 19,* 529-534. Retrieved from http://www.jultrasoundmed.org/content/19/8/529.full.pdf

Brooks, J.D., Ward, W.E., Lewis, J.E., Hilditch, J., Nickell, L., Wong, E., & Thompson, L.U. (2004) Supplementation with flaxseed alters estrogen metabolism in postmenopausal women to a greater extent than does supplementation with an equal amount of soy. *American Journal of Clinical Nutrition, 79(2),* 318-325. Retrieved from http://acjn.nutrition.org/content/79/2/318.full

Bulayeva, N., & Watson, C. (2004). Xenoestrogen-induced ERK-1 and ERK-2 activation via multiple membrane-initiated signaling pathways. *Environmental Health Perspectives, 112(15),* 1481-87. Retrieved from http://www.bvsde.paho.org/bvsacd/ehp/v112-15/p1481.pdf

Campo, S., Campo, V., & Benagiano, G. (2012). Infertility and adenomyosis. *Obstetrics and Gyneclogy International, Volume 2012,* article ID 786132. doi: 10.1155/2012/786132

Center for Endometriosis Care (2017). Adenomyosis: Is it really endometriosis? Retrieved from www.centerforendo.com/adenomyosis-is-it-really-endometriosis

Center for Endometriosis Care (2017). Excision of endometriosis. Retrieved from www.centerforendo.com/lapex-laparoscopic-excision-of-endometriosis

Center for Endometriosis Care (2017). The media got it wrong again. Retrieved from ww.centerforendometriosiscare.com/the-media-got-it-wrong-again

Cho, S., Nam, A., Kim, H., Chay, D., Park, K., Cho, D.J.,...Lee, B. (2008). Clinical effects of the levonorgesterel-releasing intrauterine device in patients with adenomyosis. *American Journal of Obstetrics and Gynecology. 198(4),* el-7. doi: 10.1016/ajog.2007.10.798

Cleveland Clinic (2018). Pelvic Floor Dysfunction. Retrieved from https://my.clevelandclinic.org/health/diseases/14459-pelvic-floor-dysfunction

Choi, E.J., Cho, S.B., Lee, S.R., Lim, Y.M., Jeong, K., Moon, H.S. & Chung, H. (2017). Comorbidity of gynecological and non-gynecological diseases with adenomyosis and endometriosis. *Obstetrics & Gynecology Science, 60(6),* 579-586. doi: 10.5468/ogs.2017.60.6.579

Cleveland Clinic (2016). Rosemary Supplement Review. Retrieved from http://www.clevelandclinicwellness.com/Features/Pages/rosemary.aspx

Covens, A.L., Christoper, R. & Casper, R.F. (1988) The effect of dietary supplementation with fish oil fatty acids on surgically induced endometriosis in the rabbit. *Fertility and Sterility, 49(4),* 698-703. Retrieved from http://www.researchgate.net/publication/20324462_The_effect_of_dietary_supplementation_with_fish_oil_fatty_acids_on_surgically_induced_endometriosis_in_the_rabbit

Cullinan-Bove, K., & Koos, R.D. (1993). Vascular endothelial growth factor/vascular permeability factor expression in the rat uterus: Rapid stimulation by estrogen correlates with estrogen-induced increases in uterine capillary permeability and growth. *Endocrinology, 133,* 829-837. http://www.ncbi.nlm.nih.gov/pubmed/8344219

Davis, S.R., Dalais, F.S., Simpson E.R. & Mukies, A.L. (1999). Phytoestrogens in health and disease. *Recent Progress in Hormone Research, 54,* 185-210, discussion 210-1. Retrieved from http://www.ncbi.nlm.nih.gov/pubmed/10548876

deSouza, N.M., Brosens, J.J., Schwieso, J.C., Paraschos, T. & Winston, R.M. (1995). The potential value of magnetic resonance imaging in infertility. *Clinical Radiology, 50(2),* 75-9. Retrieved from http://www.ncbi.nlm.nih.gov/pubmed/7867272

Deutch, B. (1995). Menstrual pain in Danish women correlated with low n-3 polyunsaturated fatty acid intake. *European Journal of Clinical Nutrition, 49(7),* 508-16. Retrieved from http://www.researchgate.net/publication/15609638_Menstrual_pain_in_Danish_women_correlated_with_low_n-3_polyunsaturated_fatty_acid_intake

Dr. Axe.com (2018). Castor Oil Speeds up Healing and Improves Your Immunity. Retrieved from https://draxe.com/castoroil/

Drugs.com (2018). Gabapentin. Retrieved from https://www.drugs.com/gabapentin.html

Drugs.com (2018). Mefenamic acid. Retrieved from https://www.drugs.com/cdi/mefenamic-acid.html

Dueholm, M., Lundorf, E., Hansen, E.S., Sorensen, J.S., Ledertoug, S., & Olesen, F. (2001). Magnetic resonance imaging and transvaginal ultrasonography for the diagnosis of adenomyosis. *Fertility and Sterility, 76,* 588-594. doi: http://dx.doi.org/10.1016/Soo15-0282(01)01962-8

Endometriosis Foundation of America. (2015). Endometriosis. Retrieved from http://www.endofound.org/endometriosis

Eubanks, M. (2004). The safety of xenoestrogens.. *Environmental Health Perspectives, 112(15),* A897. Retrieved from http://www.ncbi.nlm.nih.gov/pmc/articles/PMC1247635

Exacoustos, C., Brienza, L., DiGiovanni, A., Szaboles, B., Romanini, M.E., Supi, E. & Arduini, D. (2011). Adenomyosis: Three dimensional sonographic findings of the junctional zone and correlation with histology. *Ultrasound in Obstetrics and Gynecology, 37(4),* 471-9. doi: 10.1002/uog.8900

Fedele, L., Bianchi, S., Zonotti, F., Marchini, M., & Candiani, G.B. (1993). Fertility after conservative surgery for adenomyomas. *Human Reproduction, 8(10)*, 1708-1710. Retrieved from http://www.ncbi.nlm.nih.gov/pubmed/8300834

Focused Ultrasound Foundation. (2015). Adenomyosis. Retrieved from http://www.fusfoundation.org/diseases-and-conditions/women-s-health/adenomyosis

Fong, Y.F. & Singh, K. (1999). Medical treatment of a grossly enlarged adenomyotic uterus with the levonorgestrel-releasing intrauterine system. *Contraception, 60(3)*, 173-175. doi: 10.1016/S0010-7824(99)00075-X

Frezza, M., Tritapepe, R., Pozzato, G., & DePadova, C. (1998). Prevention of s-adenosylmethionine of estrogen-induced hepatobiliary toxicity in susceptible women. *American Journal of Gastroenterology, 83(10)*, 1098-102. Retrieved from http://www.ncbi.nlm.nih.gov/pubmed/3421220

Fry, M. (1995). Reproductive effects in birds exposed to pesticides and industrial chemicals. *Environmental Health Perspectives, 103 (Suppl 7)*, 165-171. Retrieved from http://www.ncbi.nlm.nih.gov/PMC/articles/PMC1518881/pdf/envhper00367-0160.pdf

Fukunishi, H., Funaki, K., Sawada, K., Yamaguchi, K., Tetsuo, M., & Yasushi, K. (2008). Early results of magnetic resonance-guided focused ultrasound surgery of adenomyosis: Analysis of 20 cases. *Journal of Minimally Invasive Gynecology, 15(5)*, 571-579. doi: 10.1016/j.jmig.2008.06.010

Furuhashi, M., Miyabe, Y., Katsumata, Y., Oda, H., & Imai, N. (1998). Comparison of complications of vaginal hysterectomy in patients with leiomyomas and in patients with adenomyosis. *Archives of Gynecology and Obstetrics, 262(1-2)*, 69-73. doi: 10.1007/s004040050230

Gaby, A. R. (2006). A-Z Guide to Drug-Herb-Vitamin Interactions. New York: Three Rivers Press

Ganong. W. (2003). Review of Medical Physiology. US: McGraw Hill

Garavaglia, E. Serafini, A., Inversetti, A. Ferrari, S. Tandoi, I. Corti, L. & Candiani, M. (2015). Adenomyosis and its impact on women fertility. *Iran Journal of Reproductive Medicine, 13(6)*, 327-336. Retrieved from www.ncbi.nlm.nih.gov/pubmed/?term=garavaglia+adenomyosis+and+its+impact+on+women+fertility

Garner, C. (1994). Uses of GnRH agonists. *Journal of Obstetrics and Gynecology for Neonatal Nursing, 23(7)*, 563-70. Retrieved from https://www.ncbi.nlm.nih.gov/pubmed/7996307

Gazvani, M.R., Smith, L., Haggarty, P., Fowler, P.A., & Templeton, A. (2001). High omega-3: omega-6 fatty acid ratios in culture medium reduce endometrial-cell survival in combined endometrial gland and stromal cell cultures from women with and without endometriosis. *Fertility and Sterility, 76(4)*, 717-22. Retrieved from http://www.ncbi.nlm.nih.gov/pubmed/11591404

Gehn, B., McAndrews, J., Chien, P., & Jameson, J.L. (1997). Resveratrol, a polyphenolic compound found in grapes and wine, is an agonist for the estrogen receptor. *Proceedings of the National Academy of Sciences of the United States of America, 94(25)*, 14138-14143. Retrieved from https://www.ncbi.nlm.nih.gov/pmc/articles/PMC28446/

Gilston, V. (1999). Inflammatory mediators, free radicals and gene transcription. *Progress in Inflammation Research, Feb 28*. Retrieved from www.birkhauser.ch/books/biosc/pir/pir5851toc.html

Glenza, J. (2015). Endometriosis often ignored as millions of American women suffer. *The Guardian*. Retrieved from http://www.theguardian.com/us-news/2015/sep/27/endometriosis-ignored-federal-research-funding

Goldberg, Burton. (1999). Alternative Medicine: The Definitive Guide. Tiburon: Future Medicine Publishing, Inc.

Gordts, S., Brosens, J.J., Fusi, L., Benagiano, G., & Brosens, I. (2008). Uterine adenomyosis: A need for uniform terminology and consensus classification. *Reproductive Biomedicine Online, 17(2)*, 244-8. Retrieved from http://www.ncbi.nlm.nih.gov/pubmed/18681999

Guo, S.W. (2012). Methodological issues in preclinical mouse efficacy studies of adenomyosis. *Current Obstetrics and Gynecology Reports, 1*, 138-145. doi: 10.1007/s13669-012-0018-3

Haas, Elson M. (2004). Staying Healthy with Nutrition: The Complete Guide to Diet and Nutritional Medicine. US: Celestial Arts

Harel, Z., Biro, F.M., Kottenhahn, R.K., & Rosenthal, S.L. (1996). Supplementation with omega-3 polyunsaturated fatty acids in the management of dysmenorrhea in adolescents. *American Journal of Obstetrics and Gynecology, 174(4)*, 1335-8. doi: 10.1016/S0002-9378(96)70681-6

Hayes, T., Haston, K., Tsui, M., Hoang, A., Haeffele, C., & Vonk, A. (2003). Atrazine-induced hermaphroditism at 0.1 ppb in American leopard frogs (Ranna pipiens): Laboratory and field evidence. *Environmental Health Perspectives, 111(4),* 568-575. Retrieved from http://www.ncbi.nlm. nih.gov/pubmed/PMC1241446

Hirata, T., Izumi, G., Takamura, M., Saito, A., Nakazawa, A., Harada, M.,...Osuga, Y. (2014). Efficacy of dienogest in the treatment of symptomatic adenomyosis: A pilot study. *Gynecology and Endocrinology,* 1-4. Retrieved from http://www.ncbi.nlm.nih.gov/pubmed/24905725

Hiroyuki, M., Ideda, T., Kajita, K., Fujioka, K., Mori, L., Okada, H.,...Ishizuka, T. (2012). Effect of royal jelly ingestion for six months on healthy volunteers. *Nutrition Journal, 11,* 77. doi: 10.1186/1475-2891-11-77

Huang, W.H., Yang, T.S., & Yuan, C.C. (1998). Successful pregnancy after treatment of deep adenomyosis with cytoreductive surgery and subsequent gonadotropin-releasing hormone agonist: A case report. *Zhonghua Yi Xue Za Zhi, 61(12),* 726-9. Retrieved from http://www.ncbi.nlm.nih.gov/pubmed/ 9884446

Humphrey, C.D. (1998). Phytoestrogens and human health effects: Weighing up the current evidence. *Natural Toxins, 6(2),* 51-9. Retrieved from http:// www.ncbi.nlm.nih.gov/pubmed/98886300

Hyder, S.M., Nawaz, Z., Chiappetta, C., & Stancel, G.M. (2000). Identification of functional estrogen response elements in the gene coding for the potent angiogenic factor vascular endothelial growth factor. *Cancer Research, 60,* 3183-3190. Retrieved from www.ncbi.nlm.nih.gov/pubmed/?term=hyder+ identification+of+functional+estrogen+response+elements

Interstitial Cystitis Foundation (2018). Pelvic floor dysfunction. Retrieved from https://www.ichelp.org/about-ic/associated-conditions/pelvic-floor-dysfuction/

Jabr, F.I., & Mani, V. (2014). An unusual case of abdominal pain in a male patient: Endometriosis. *Avicenna Journal of Medicine, 4(4),* 99-101. doi:10.4103/2231-0770.140660

Jackson-Michel, S. (2015). Herbs for estrogen dominance. Retrieved from http://www.livestrong.com/article/123225-herbs-estrogen-dominance

Jefferson, W.N., Padilla-Banks, E., & Newbold, R.R. (2007). Disruption of the developing female reproductive system by phytoestrogens: Genistein as an example. *Molecular Nutrition and Food Research, 51(7),* 832-844. doi: 10.1002/mnfr.200600258

Jenkinson, P.C., Anderson, D., & Gangollli, S.D. (1986). Malformations induced in cultured rat embryos by enzymically generated active oxygen species. *Teratogenesis, Carcinogenesis and Mutagenesis, 6,* 547-54. Retrieved from www.ncbi.nlm.nih.gov/pubmed/?term=jenkinson+malformations+induced+in +cultured+rat+embryos

Johns Hopkins Medicine (2018). Endometrial biopsy. Retrieved from https:// hopkinsmedicine.org/healthlibrary/test_procedures/gynecology/endometrial_ biopsy_92.PO773

Johns Hopkins Medicine (2018). Pelvic congestion syndrome. Retrieved from http://www.hopkinsmedicine.org/interventional-radiology/conditions/ pelvic/index.html

Johns Hopkins Medicine (2018). Polycystic Ovarian Syndrome (PCOS). Retrieved from https://www.hopkinsmedicine.org/healthlibrary/conditions/ adult/endocrinology/polycystic_ovarian_syndrome_PCOS_85.PO8334

Johnson, J. (2017). Everything you need to know about CBD oil. Medical News Today. Retrieved from www.medicalnewstoday.com/articles/317221.php

Johnston, I.M. & Johnston, J.R. (1990). Flaxseed (Linseed) Oil and the Power of Omega-3. US: Keats Publishing.

Jung, B.I., Kin, M.S., Kim, H.A., Kim D., Yang, J., Her, S., & Song, Y.S. (2010). Caffeic acid phenethylester, a component of beehive propolis, is a novel selective estrogen receptor modulator. *Phytotherapy Research, 24(2),* 295-300. doi: 10.1002/ptr.2966

Justis, A. (2018). Raspberry leaf benefits for women. The Herbal Academy. Retrieved from https://theherbalacademy.com/3-raspberry-leaf-benefits-for-women/

Kaplan, J.M., Cook, J.A., Hake, P.W., O'Conner, M., Burroughs, T. J. & Zingarelli, B. (2005). 15-deoxy-delta(12,14)-prostaglandin J(2) (15D-PGJ(2)), a peroxisome proliferator activated receptor gamma ligand, reduces tissue leucosequestration and mortality in endotoxic shock. *Shock, Jul; 24(1),* 59-65. Retrieved from www.ncbi.nlm.nih.gov/pubmed/15988322

Kaye, J. (2011). Xenoestrogens. Retrieved from http://www.drjosephkaye. com/2011/10/14/xenoestrogens/

Khanaki, K., Nouri, M., Ardekani, A.M., Ghassemzadeh, A., Shahnazi, V., Sadeqhi, M.R.,…Rahimipour, A. (2012). Evaluation of the relationship between endometriosis and omega-3 and omega-6 polyunsaturated fatty acids. *Iranian Biomedical Journal, 16(1),* 38-43. doi: 10.6091/IBJ.10.25.2012

Kijma, L., Phung, S., Hur, G., Kwok, S.L., & Chen,S. (2006). Grape seed extract is an aromatase inhibitor and a suppressor of aromatase expression. *Cancer Research, 66(11),* 5960-7. Retrieved from http://www.ncbi.nlm.nih.gov/pubmed/16740737

Kim, K.A., Yoon, S.W., Lee, C., Seong, S.J., Yoon, B.S., & Park, H. (2011). Short-term results of magnetic resonance imaging-guided focused ultrasound surgery for patients with adenomyosis: Symptomatic relief and pain reduction. *Fertility and Sterility, 95(3),* 1152-1155. doi: 10.1016/j.fertandstert. 2010.09.024

Kim, M.J., Park, J.H., Kwon, D.Y., Yang, H.J., Kim da, S., Kang, S., & Park, S. (2014). The supplementation of Korean mistletoe water extracts reduces hot flushes, dyslipidemia, hepatic steatosis, and muscle loss in ovariectomized rats. *Experimental Biology and Medicine, 240(4),* 477-87. doi: 10.1177/1535370214551693

Kimura, F., Takahashi, K., Takebayashi, K., Fujiwara, M., Kita, N., Noda, Y.,…Harada, N. (2007). Concomitant treatment of severe uterine adenomyosis in a premenopausal woman with an aromatase inhibitor and a gonadotropin-releasing hormone agonist. *Fertility and Sterility, 87.* Retrieved from www.ncbi.nlm.nih.gov/pubmed/17222833

King, M. (2003). Biochemistry of neurotransmitters. IU School of Medicine. Retrieved from http://www.indstate.edu/theme/mwking/nerves.html

Kunisue, T., Chen, Z., Buck Louis, G., Sundaram, R., Hediger, M., Sun, L., & Kannan, K. (2012). Urinary concentrations of benzophenone-type UV filters in US women and their association with endometriosis. *Environmental Science and Technology, 46(8),* 4624-4632. doi: 10.1021/es204415a

Kunz, G., Herbertz, M., Beil, D., Huppert, P., & Leyendecker, G. (2007). Adenomyosis as a disorder of the early and late human reproductive period. *Reproductive Biomedicine Online, 15(6),* 681-5. Retrieved from http://ncbi.nlm.nih.gov/pubmed/18062865

Kurzer, M.S. (2002). Hormonal effects of soy in premenopausal women and men. *Journal of Nutrition, 132(3),* 570S-573S. Retrieved from http://www.ncbi.nlm.nih.gov/pubmed/11880595

Lam, M. (2015a). Estrogen dominance – Part 1. Retrieved from http://www.drlam/com/Articles/Estrogen_Dominance.asp

Lam, M. (2015b). Estrogen dominance – Part 2. Retrieved from http://www.drlam.com/blog/estrogen-dominance-part-2/1781/

Lam, M. (2015c). How and when did estrogen dominance arise? Retrieved from http://ww.biomediclabs.com/health-articles/

LaRue, A. (2012). Xenoestrogens – What are they? How to avoid them. Women in Balance Institute: National College of Natural Medicine. Retrieved from http://womeninbalance.org/2012/10/26/xenoestrogens-what-are-they-how-to-avoid-them/

Lee,J.R. (2016). Four simple steps for balancing hormones naturally. Retrieved from http://www.johnleemd.com

Lee, J. R. and Hopkins, V. (2004). What Your Doctor May Not Tell You About Menopause: The Breakthrough Book on Natural Hormone Balance. US: Hatchett Book Group.

Lee, S.R., Yi, K.W., Song, J.Y., Seo, S.K., Lu, D.Y., Cho, S., & Kim, S.H. (2017). Efficacy and safety of long-term use of dienogest in women with ovarian endometrioma. *Reproductive Sciences, Jan 1*:1933719117725820. doi: 10.1177/ 1933719117725820

Leonetti, H.B., Wilson, K.J., & Anasti, J.N. (2003). Topical progesterone cream has an antiproliferative effect on estrogen-stimulated endometrium. *Fertility and Sterility, 79(1),* 221-222. Retrieved from www.fertstert.org/ article/S0015-0282(02)04542-9/fulltext

Leyendecker,G., Kunz, G., Wildt, L., Beil, D., & Deiinger, H. (1996). Uterine hyperperistalsis and dysperistalsis as dysfunctions of the mechanism of rapid sperm transport in patients with endometriosis and infertility. *Human Reproduction, 11(7),* 1542-51. Retrieved from http://www.ncbi.nlm.nih.gov/ pubmed/8671502

Leyendecker, G., Wildt, L. & Mall, G. The pathophysiology of endometriosis and adenomyosis: Tissue injury and repair. *Archives of Gynecology and Obstetrics, 280,* 529-538. doi: 10.1007/s00404-009-1191-0

Li, H., Liu, D. & Zhang, E. (2000). Effect of fish oil supplementation on fatty acid composition and neurotransmitters of growing rats. *Wei Sheng Yan Jiu, 29(1).* Retrieved from www.ncbi.nlm.nih.gov/entrez/query.fcgi?cmd=Retrieve&db =PubMed&list_uids=12725043&dopt=Abstract

Lin, J., Sun, C., & Li, R. (1999). Gonadotropin releasing hormone agonists in the treatment of adenomyosis with infertility. *Zhonghua Fu Chan Ke Za Zhi, 34(4),* 214-16. Retrieved from http://www.ncbi.nlm.nih.gov/pubmed/11326917

Linus Pauling Institute (2015). Resveratrol. Retrieved from www.lpi. oregonstate.edu/mic/dietary-factors/phytochemicals/resveratrol

Lipski, E. (2000). Digestive Wellness. US: Keats Publishing

Liske, E., Hanggi, M.D., & Henneicke-von Zepelin, H.H. (2002). Physiological investigation of a unique extract of black cohosh (cimicfugae racemosae rhizome): A 6-month clinical study demonstrates no systemic estrogenic effect. *Journal of Women's Health & Gender-Based Medicine, 11,* 163-174. Retrieved from http://www.ncbi.nlm.nih.gov/pubmed/11975864

Liu, J., Burdette, J.E., & Xu, H. (2001). Evaluation of estrogenic activity of plant extracts for the potential treatment of menopausal symptoms. *Journal of Agricultural and Food Chemistry, 49,* 2472-2479. Retrieved from http://www.ncbi.nlm.nih.gov/pubmed/11368622

Liu, J.J., Duan, H., & Wang, S. (2013). Expression of nitric oxide in uterine junctional zone of patients with adenomyosis. *Zhonghua Fu Chan Ke Za Shi, 48(7),* 504-7. Retrieved from http://www.ncbi.nlm.nih.gov/pubmed/24284220

LiveLifeRenewed.com (2004). Fats and Oils. Retrieved from www. liverenewedlife.com/fats_oils.html

Loffer, F. D. (1995). Endometrial ablation and resection. *Current Opinion in Obstetrics and Gynecology, 7(4),* 290-4. Retrieved from http://www.ncbi. nlm.nih.gov/pubmed/7578969

Luukkainen, T., Toivonen, J., & Pakarinen, P. (2002). Progestin-releasing intrauterine systems. *Seminars in Reproductive Medicine, 19(4),* 355-63. doi: 10.1055/s-2001-18643

Mabey, R. (1988). The New Age Herbalist. US: Simon and Schuster

Machida, T., Taga, M. & Minaguchi, H. (1997). Prolactin secretion in endometriotic patients. *European Journal of Obstetrics and Gynecology and Reproductive Biology, 72,* 89-92. Retrieved from http://www.ncbi. nlm.nih.gov/pubmed/9076428

Mansukhani, N., Unni, J., Dua, M., Darbari, R., Malik, S., Verma, S., & Bathla, S. (2013). Are women satisfied when using levonorgestrel-releasing uterine system for treatment of abnormal uterine bleeding? *Journal of Mid-Life Health, 4(1),* 31-35. doi: 10.4103/0976-78--.109633

Martin, J.D. & Hauck, H.E. (1985). Endometriosis in the male. *American Journal of Surgery, 51(7),* 426-30. Retrieved from http://www.ncbi.nlm.nih.gov/pubmed/4014886

Marvibaigi, M., Supriyanto, E., Amini, N., Majid, F.A.A., & Jaganathan, S.K. (2014). Preclinical and clinical effects of mistletoes against breast cancer. *BioMed Research International, Volume 2014,* article ID 785479. doi: 10.1155/2014/785479

Mayo Clinic (2018). Ovarian cysts. Retrieved from www.mayoclinic.org/diseases-conditions/ovarian-cysts/symptoms-causes/syc-20353405

Mehasseb, M.K. & Habiba, M.S. (2009). Adenomyosis uteri: An update. *The Obstetrician and Gynaecologist, 11,* 41-47. doi: 10.1576/toag.11.1.41/27467

Mendes da Silva, D., Gross, L.A., Neto, E.P.G., Lessey, B.A., & Savaris, R.F. (2017). The use of resveratrol as an adjuvant treatment of pain in endometriosis: A randomized clinical trial. *Journal of the Endocrine Society, 1(4),* 359-369. doi: 10.1210/js.2017-00053

Meredith, S.M., Sanchez-Ramos, L., & Kaunitz, A.M. (2009). Diagnostic accuracy of transvaginal sonography for the diagnosis of adenomyosis: Systemic review and meta-analysis. *American Journal of Obstetrics and Gynecology, 201,* 107, e1-6. doi: 10.1016/j.ajog.2009.03.021

Millischer, A., Borghese, B., Santulli, P. Lecomte, M., Cousset, B., & Capron, C. (2013). Could adenomyosis be considered as a marker of severity in intestinal endometriosis? *Ultrasound in Obstetrics and Gynecology, 42,* 4. doi: 10.1002/uog.12590

Missmer, S.A., Chavarro, J.E., Malspeis, S., Bertone-Johnson, E.R., & Hornstein, M.D. (2010). A prospective study of dietary fat consumption and endometriosis risk. *Human Reproduction, 25(6),* 1528-35. doi: 10.1093/humrep/deq044

Molinas, C.R., & Campo, R. (2006). Office hysteroscopy and adenomyosis. *Best Practices and Research Clinical Obstetrics and Gynaecology, 20(4),* 557-67. Retrieved from http://www.ncbi.nlm.nih.gov/pubmed/16554185

Moore, R.W., Rudy, T.A., Lin, T.M., Ko, K., & Peterson, R.E. (2001). Abnormalities of sexual development in male rats with in utero and lactational exposure to the antiandrogenic plasticizer di(2-ethyl(hexyl)phthalate.

Environmental Health Perspectives, 109(3), 229-237. Retrieved from
http://www.ncbi.nlm.nih.gov/pmc/articles/PMC1240240

Mori, T., Singtripop, T., & Kawashima, S. (1991). Animal model of uterine
adenomyosis: Is prolactin a potent inducer of adenomyosis in mice? *American
Journal of Obstetrics and Gynecology, 165(1),* 232-4. Retrieved from https://
www.ncbi.nlm.nih.gov/pubmed/1853904

Morohoshi, K., Yamamoto, H., Kamata, R., Shiraishi, F. Koda T., & Morita, M.
(2005). Estrogenic activity of 37 components of commercial sunscreen lotions
evaluated by in vitro assays. *Journal of Toxicology In Vitro, (19), 4,* 457-69. doi:
10.1016/j.tiv.2005.01.004

National Institutes of Health. (2016). Black cohosh. Retrieved from http://oda.
od.nih.gov/factsheets/BlackCohosh-HealthProfessional/

Noda, Y., Matsumoto, H., Umaoka, Y., Tatsumi, K., Kishi, J., & Mori, T. (1991).
Involvement of superoxide radicals in the mouse two-cell block. *Molecular
Reproduction and Development, 28(4),* 356-60. Retrieved from http://www.
ncbi.nlm.nih.gov/pubmed/1648368

Northrup, C. (2016). Estrogen Dominance. Retrieved from http://www.
drnorthrup.com/estrogen-dominance/

Novellas, S., Chassang, M., Delotte, J., Toullalan, O., Chevallier, A., Boouasis, J.,
& Chevalier, P. (2011). MRI characteristics of the uterine junctional zone: From
normal to the diagnosis of adenomyosis. *American Journal of Roentgenology,
196(5).* doi: 10.2214/AJR.10.4877

Null, G. (1997). Healing Your Body Naturally: Alternative Treatments to Illness.
US: Seven Stories.

Ochoa-Maya, M.R. (2012). Treatment considerations for excess estrogen and
estrogen dominance. Freedom to Heal. Retrieved from http://www.
freedomtoheal.org/2012/08/treatment-considerations-for-excess.html

Oh, S.J., Shin, J.H., Kim, T.H., Lee, H.S., Yoo, J.Y., Ahn, J.Y.,...Jeong, J.W. (2013).
B-catenin activation contributes to the pathogenesis of adenomyosis through
epithelial-mesenchymal transition. *Journal of Pathology, 231(2),* 210-222. doi:
10.1002/path.4224

Osada, H., Silberb, S., Kakinuma, T., Nagaishia, M., Katoc, K., & Katoc, O.
(2010). Surgical procedure to conserve the uterus for future pregnancy in
patients suffering from massive adenomyosis. *Reproductive BioMedicine*

Online. Retrieved from http://www.infertile.com/inthenew/sci/2010-09-RBMO-adenomyosis.htm

Ota, H., Igarashi, S., Hatazawa, J., & Tanaka, T. (1998). Is adenomyosis an immune disease? *Human Reproduction Update, 4(4),* 360-7. Retrieved from http://www.ncbi.nlm.nih.gov/pubmed/9825851

Ota, H., Igarashi, S., Hatazawa, J., & Tanaka, T. (1998). Endothelial nitric oxide synthase in the endometrium during the menstrual cycle in patients with endometriosis and adenomyosis. *Fertility and Sterility, 69,* 303-308. Retrieved from http://www.ncbi.nlm.nih.gov/m/pubmed/9496346

Overk, C.R., Yao, P., Chadwick, L.R., Nikolic, D., Sun, Y., Cuendet, M.A.,...Bolton, J.L. (2005). Comparison of the in vitro estrogenic activities of compounds from hops (humulus lupulus) and red clover (trifolium pretense). *Journal of Agriculture and Food Chemistry, 53(16),* 6246-53. Retrieved from http://ncbi.nlm.nih.gov/pubmed/16076101

Owalbi, T.O., & Strickler, R.C. (1977). Adenomyosis: A neglected diagnosis. *Obstetrics and Gynecology, 50(4),* 424-7. Retrieved from www.ncbi.nlm.nih.gov/pubmed/904805

Pagedas, A.C., Bae, I.H., & Perkins, H.E. (1995). Review of 24 cases of uterine ablation failure. *Journal of Minimally Invasive Gynecology, 2(4),* S39. doi: 10.1016/S1074-3804(05)80588-2

Panganamamula, U.R., Harmanli, O.H., Isik-Akbay, E.F., Grotegut, C.A., Dandolu, V., & Gaughan, J.P. (2004). Is prior uterine surgery a risk factor for adenomyosis? *Obstetrics and Gynecology, 104(5),* 1034-1038. doi: 10.1097/01.AOG.0000143264.59822.73

Parazzini, F., Vercellini, P., Panazza, S., Chatenoud, L., Oldani, S., & Crosignani, P. (1997). Risk factors for adenomyosis. *Human Reproduction, 12(6),* 1275-1279. Retrieved from http://www.humrep.oxfordjournals.org/Content/12/6/1275.full.pdf

Parazzini, F., Paola,V., Candiani, M., & Fedele, L. (2013). Diet and endometriosis risk: A literature review. *Reproductive BioMedicine Online, 26(4),* 323-336. doi: 10.1016/j.rbmo.2012.12.011

Parker, J.D., Leondires, M., Sinaii, N., Premkumar, A., Nieman, L.K., & Stratton, P. (2006). Persistence of dysmenorrhea and nonmenstrual pain after optimal endometriosis surgery may indicate adenomyosis. *Fertility and Sterility, 86(3),* 711-715. doi: 10.1016/j.fertnstert.2006.01.030

Patisaul, H. & Jefferson, W. (2010). The pros and cons of phytoestrogens. *Frontiers in Neuroendocrinology, 31(4),* 400-419. doi: 10.1016/i.vfrne. 2010.03.003

Peat, R. (2014). Progesterone, pregnenolone & DHEA – Three youth-associated hormones. Retrieved from http://raypeat.com/articles/articles/three-hormones.shtml

Pederson, Mark (1998). Nutritional Herbology: A Reference Guide to Herbs. US: Wendell W. Whitman Company

Pelage, J.P., Jacob, D., Fazel, A., Namur, J., Laurent, A., Rymer, R., & LeDref, O. (2005). Midterm results of uterine artery embolization for symptomatic adenomyosis: Initial experience. *Vascular and Interventional Radiology, 234 (3).* doi: 10.1148/radiol.2343031697

Peng, Y.H., Su, S.Y., Liao, W.C., Huang, C.W., Hsu, C.Y., Chen, H.J....Wu, C.C. (2017). Asthma is associated with endometriosis: A retrospective population-based cohort study. *Respiratory Medicine, 132,* 112-116. doi: 10.1016/jrmed.2017.10.004

Pick, M. (2013). Is It Me or My Hormones? US: Hay House, Inc.

Plymate, S.R., Matei, L.A., Jones, R.E., & Freidl, K.E. (1988). Inhibition of sex hormone-binding globulin production in the human hepatoma (Hep-G2) cell line by insulin and prolactin. *The Journal of Clinical Endocrinology & Metabolism, 67(3),* 460-4. Retrieved from https://www.ncbi.nlm.nih.gov/pubmed/2842359

Powers, C.N. & Setzer, W.N. (2015). A molecular docking study of phytochemical estrogen mimics from dietary herbal supplements. *In Silico Pharmacology, 3,* 4. doi: 10.1186/s40203-015-0008-z

Pressman, A. & Buff, S. (2000). The Complete Idiots Guide to Vitamins and Minerals. US: Alpha Books

Prior, J.C., Vigna, Y.M., & McKay, D.W. (1992). Reproduction for the athletic woman. New understandings of physiology and management. *Sports Medicine, 14(3),* 190-9. Retrieved from www.ncbi.nlm.nih.gov/pubmed/1439394

Rank, A. (2004). Eicosanoids. Wake Forest University. Retrieved from http://www.wfu.edu/users/clafme0/nutrition/eicosanoids.html

Rato, A.G., Pedrero, J.G., Martinez, M.A., Rio, B.D., Lazo, P.D., & Ramos, S. (1999). Melatonin blocks the activation of estrogen receptor for DNA binding. *FASEB Journal, 13(8)*, 857-868. Retrieved from http://www.fasebj.org/content/13/8/857.full

Rebbeck, T.R., Troxel, A.B., Norman, S., Bunin, G.R., DeMichele, A., Baumgarten, M.,...Strom, B.L. (2007). A retrospective case-control study of the use of hormone-related supplements and association with breast cancer. *International Journal of Cancer, 120*, 1523-1528. doi: 10.1002/ijc.22485

Redwine, D. (2006). Complications of LUNA and presacral neurectomy by laparoscopy. Retrieved from www.laparoscopy.blogs.com/prevention-management/Chapter_23_lunapresacral_neurectomy/

Reinhold, C., McCarthy, S., Bret, P.M., Mehio, A., Atri, M., Zakarian, R.,...Seymour, R.J. (1996). Diffuse adenomyosis: Comparison of endovaginal US and MR imaging with histopathologic correlation. *Radiology, 199(1)*, 151-8. Retrieved from http://www.ncbi.nlm.nih.gov/pubmed/8633139

Rocha, A.L.L., Reis, F., & Taylor, R. (2013). Angiogenesis and endometriosis. *Obstetrics and Gynecology International, 2013*, Article ID 859619. doi: 10.1155/2013/8596119

Rudin, D. & Felix, C. (1996). Omega-3 Oils, A Practical Guide. US: Avery

Safirstein, A. (2015). Estrogen Dominance. Retrieved from http://fromcancertohealth.com/estrogen-dominance/

Schliep, K.C., Schisterman,E.F., Mumford, S.L., Pollack,A.Z., Zang, C., Ye, A.,...Wactawshi-Wende, J. (2012). Caffeinated beverage intake and reproductive hormones among premenopausal women in the biocycle study. *The American Journal of Clinical Nutrition, 95(2)*, 488-497. doi: 10.3954/acjn.111.021287

Schlumpf, M., Durrer, S., Faass, O., Ehnes, C., Fuetsch, M., Gaille, C.,...Lichtensteiger, W. (2008). Developmental toxicity of UV filters and environmental exposure: A review. *International Journal of Andrology, 31(2)*, 144-51. doi: 10.1111/j.1365-2605.2007.00856.x

Sears, B. (2002). The Omega Rx Zone: The Miracle of the New High-Dose Fish Oil. US: Harper Collins Publishers, Inc.

Seidl, M.M. & Stewart, D.C. (1998). Alternative treatments for menopausal symptoms: Systematic review of scientific and lay literature. *Canadian Family*

Physician, volume 44. Retrieved from http://www.europepmc.org/backend/ptpmcrender.fcgi?accid=PMC2278270&blobtype=pdf

Sengupta, P., Sharma, A., Mazumdar, G., Banerjee, I., Tripathi, S., Bagchi, C., & Das, N. (2013). The possible role of fluoxetine in adenomyosis: An animal experiment with clinical correlations. *Journal of Clinical and Diagnostic Research, 7(7),* 1530-1534. doi: 10.7860/JCDR/2013/5654.3128

Sheng, J., Zhang, W.Y., Zhang, J.P. & Lu, D. (2009). The LNS-IUS study on adenomyosis: A 3-year follow-up study on the efficacy and side effects of the use of levonorgestrel intrauterine system for the treatment of dysmenorrhea associated with adenomyosis. *Contraception, 79(3),* 189-93. doi: 10.1016/j.contraception.2008.11.004

Sheth, S.S., & Ray, S.S. (2014). Severe adenomyosis and CA125. *Journal of Obstetrics and Gynaecology, 34(1),* 79-81. doi: 10.3109/01443615.2013.832178

Shier, D., Butler, J., & Lewis. R. (1996). Hole's Human Anatomy and Physiology. US: The McGraw Hill Companies, Inc.

Shrestha, A. & Sedai, L.B. (2012). Understanding clinical features of adenomyosis: A case control study. *Nepal Medical College Journal, 14(3),* 176-9. Retrieved from http://www.ncbi.nlm.nih.gov/pubmed/24047010

Shweiki, D. Itin, A., Neufeld, G., Gitay-Goren, H. & Keshet, E. (1993). Patterns of expression of vascular endothelial growth factor (VEGF) and VEGF receptors in mice suggest a role in hormonally regulated angiogenesis. *Journal of Clinical Investigation, 91,* 2235-2243. Retrieved from http://www.ncbi.nlm.nih.gov/pubmed/7683699

Simopoulos, A.P. (2000). Evolutionary aspects of diet and essential fatty acids. Kronos Institute Seminar Series. Retrieved from http://kronosinstitute.org/seminars/seminar-2000-10-31-simopoulos.html

Simopoulos, A.P. (2003). Omega-3 fatty acids in inflammation and autoimmune diseases. *Journal of the American College of Nutrition, 21(6).* Retrieved from http://www.ncbi.nlm.nih.gov/entrez/query.fcgi?cmd=retrieve&db=PubMed&list_uids=12480795&dopt=Abstract

Sinatra, S., Sinatra, J., & Lieberman R.J. (2001). Heart Sense for Women. US: Penguin Putnam, Inc.

Sinervo, K. (2017). Endometriosis and Bowel Symptoms. Center for Endometriosis Care. Retrieved from www.centerforendo.com/endometriosis-and-bowel-symptoms

Sinervo, K. (2018). Presacral Neurectomy. Center for Endometriosis Care. Retrieved from: www.centerforendo.com/presacral-neurectomy/

Siskin, G.P., Tublin, M.E., Stainken, B.F., Dowling, K. & Dolen, E.G. (2001). Uterine artery embolization for the treatment of adenomyosis: Clinical response and evaluation with MR imaging. *American Journal of Roentgenology, 177(2),* 297-302. Retrieved from http://www.ncbi.nlm.nih.gov/pubmed/ 11461849

Slomczynska, M. (2008). Xenoestrogens: Mechanisms of action and some detection studies. *Polish Journal of Veterinary Sciences, 11(3),* 263-9. Retrieved from http://www.ncbi.nlm.nih.gov/pubmed/18942551

Smith, E. (2004). Adenomyosis. Retrieved from http;//www.adeno101.com/

Smith, E. (2014). How to avoid xenoestrogens that cause adenomyosis. Retrieved from http://www.adeno101.com/xeno.htm

Smith, P.W. (2010). What You Must Know About Women's Hormones: Your Guide to Natural Hormone Treatments for PMS, Menopause, Osteoporosis, PCOS and More. US: Square One Publishers

Soysal, S., Soysal, M.E., Ozer, S., Gul, N. & Gezgin, T. (2004). The effects of post-surgical administration of goserelin plus anastrozole compared to goserelin alone in patients with severe endometriosis: A prospective randomized trial. *Human Reproduction, 19(1),* 160. doi: 10.1093/humanrep/ deh035

Streuli, I., Dubuisson, J., Santulli, P., de Ziegler, D., Batteux, F. & Chapron, C. (2014). An update on the pharmacological management of adenomyosis. *Expert Opinion on Pharmacotherapy, 15(16),* 2347-2360. doi: 10.1517/ 14656566.2014.953055

Tao, J., Zhang, P., Liu, G., Yan, H., Bu, X., Ma, Z.,...Lia, W. (2009). Cytotoxicity of Chinese motherwort (yimucao) aqueous ethanol extract is non-apoptotic and estrogen receptor independent on human breast cancer cells. *Journal of Ethnopharmacology, 122(2),* 234-9. Retrieved from http://www.ncbi.nlm.nih.gov/pubmed/19330917

Taran, F.A., Weaver, A.L., Coddington, C.C. & Stewart, E.A. (2010). Understanding adenomyosis: A case control study. *Fertility and Sterility, 94(4),* 1223-8. doi: 10.1016/j.fertnstert.2009.06.049

Taran, F.A., Stewart, E.A. & Brucker, S. (2013). Adenomyosis: Epidemiology, risk factors, clinical phenotype and surgical and interventional alternatives to hysterectomy. *Geburtshife Frauenheilkd, 73(9),* 924-931. doi: 10.1055/s-0033-1350840

Taylor, H.S. (2000). The role of HOX genes in human implantation. *Human Reproduction Update, 6(1),* 75-9. Retrieved from http://www.ncbi.nlm.nih.gov/pubmed/10711832

The Dr. Oz Show. (2015). Soy: The good, the bad and the best. Retrieved from http://www.doctoroz.com/print/45041

Thompson, J.F. (2016). Exam 5 Review: Chapter 27 Uterine Anatomy. In Austin Peay State University Biology Website. Retrieved from www.apsubiology.org/anatomy/2020.2020_Exam_Reviews/Exam_s/CH27_Uterine_Anatomy.htm

Tokyol, C., Aktepe, F., Dilek, F.H., Sahin, O. & Arioz, D.T. (2009). Expression of cyclooxygenase-2 and matrix metalloproteinase-2 in adenomyosis and endometrial polyps and its correlation with angiogenesis. *International Journal of Gynecological Pathology, 28(2),* 148-56. doi: 10.1097/PGP.0b013e318187033b

Tomio, K., Kawana K., Taguchi, A., Isobe, Y., Iwamoto, R., Yamashita, A.,...Kojima, S. (2013). Omega-3 polyunsaturated fatty acids suppress the cystic lesion formation of peritoneal endometriosis in transgenic mouse models. *PLoS ONE, 8(9),* e73085. doi: 10.1371/journal.pone.0073085

University of Maryland Medical Center (2001). Omega-6 fatty acids. Retrieved from http://www.umm.edu/altmed/ConsSupplements/Omega6FattyAcidscs.html

University of Maryland Medical Center (2016). Evening primrose oil (EPO). In Complementary and Alternative Medicine Guide – Herbs. Retrieved from http://www.umm.edu/health/medical/altmed/herb/evening-primrose-oil

University of Michigan Medicine (2018). Pregnenolone. Retrieved from www.uofmhealth.org/health-library/hn-2899008

Upson, K., DeRoos, A.J., Thompson, M.L., Sathyanarayana, S., Scholes, D., Barr, D.B. & Holt, V.L. (2013). Organochlorine pesticides and risk of endometriosis:

Finding from a population-based case-control study. *Environmental Health Perspectives, 121,* 11-12. doi: 10.1289/ehp.1306648

Urologyhealth.org (2017). Interstitial cystitis. Retrieved from http://www.urologyhealth.org/urological-conditions/interstitial-cystitis/treatment

Van der Woulde, H., Ter Veld, M.G., Jacobs, N., van der Saag, P.T., Murk, A.J. & Rietjens, I.M. (2005). The stimulation of cell proliferation by quercetin is mediated by the estrogen receptor. *Molecular Nutrition and Food Research, 49(8),* 763-71. Retrieved from http://www.ncbi.nlm.nih.gov/pubmed/15937998

Vercellini, P., Consonni, D., Dridi, D., Bracco, B., Frattaruolo, M.P. & Somigliana, E. (2014). Uterine adenomyosis and in vitro fertilization outcome: A systematic review and meta-analysis. *Human Reproduction, 29(5),* 964-77. Retrieved from http://www.unboundmedicine.com/medline/citation/24622619/Uterine_adenomyosis_and_in_vitro_fertilization_outcome:a_systematic_review_and_meta_analysis

Vermesh, M., Fossum, G.T., & Kletzky, O. (1988). Vaginal bromocriptine: Pharmacology and effect on serum prolactin in normal women. *Obstetrics and Gynecology.* Retrieved from https://journals.lww.com/greenjournal/Abstract/1988/11000/Vaginal_Bromocriptine_Pharmacology_and_Effect_on.3.aspx

Viñas, R. & Watson, C. (2013). Mixtures of xenoestrogens disrupt estradiol-induced non-genomic signaling and downstream functions in pituitary cells. *Environmental Health Perspective, 12,* 26. doi: 10.1186/1476-069X-12-26

Walsh, B. (2011). Study: Even 'BPA-free' plastics leach endocrine-disrupting chemicals. *Time.* Retrieved 14 September 2016.

Wang, F., Li, H., Yang, Z., Du, X., Cui, M., & Wen, Z. (2009). Expression of interleukin-10 in patients with adenomyosis. *Fertility and Sterility, 91,* 1681-1685. doi: 10.1016/j.fertnstert/2008.02.164

Wang, H.S., Tsai, C.L., Chang, P.Y., Chao, A., Wu, R.C., Chen, S.H.,...Wang, T.H. (2018). Positive associations between upregulated levels of stress-induced phosphoprotein1 and matrix metalloproteinase-9 in endometriois/adenomyosis. *PLoS One, 13(1),* e0190573. doi: 10.1371/ journal.pone.0190573

Wang, J., Zhang, H.H. & Duan H. (2010). Expression of ERα in endometrial-myometrial interface of human adenomyosis. *Zhonghua Yi Xue Za Zhi, 90(27),* 1914-17. Retrieved from http://www.ncbi.nlm.nih.gov/pubmed/20979911

WebMD.com (2016). Anise. In Vitamins and Supplements. Retrieved from http://www.webmd.com/vitamins-supplements/ingredientmono-582-anise.aspx?activeingredientid=582&acitveingredientname=anise

WebMD.com (2016). Indole-3-carbinol. In Vitamins and Supplements. Retrieved from http://www.webmd.com/vitamins-supplements/ingredientmono-1027-indole-3-carbinol.aspx?activeingredientid=1027&activeingredientname=indole-3-carbinol

WebMD.com (2016). Licorice. In Vitamins and Supplements. Retrieved from http://www.webmd.com/vitamins-supplements/ingredientmono-881-LICORICE.aspx?activeingredientid=881&activeingredientname=LICORICE

WebMD.com (2016). Pyridoxine (vitamin B6). In Vitamins and Supplements. Retrieved from http://www.webmd.com/vitamins-supplements/ingredient mono-934-pyridoxine%20vitamin%20b6.aspx?activeingredientid=934&active ingredientname=pyridoxine

WebMD.com (2016). Thyme. In Vitamins and Supplements. Retrieved from http://www.webmd.com/vitamins-supplements/ingredientmono-823-thyme.aspx?activeingredient=823&activeingredientname=thyme

WebMD.com (2016). Turmeric. In Vitamins and Supplements. Retrieved from http://www.webmd.com/vitamins-supplements/ingredientmono-662-turmeric.aspx?activeingredient=662&activeingredientname=turmeric

Weil, A. (2000). Eating Well for Optimum Health. US: Alfred A. Knopf

WholeHealthMD.com (2005). Chasteberry. In Supplements. Retrieved from http://www.wholehealthmd.com/ME2/dirmod.asp?type=AWHN-Supplements&tier=2&id=B876FF3FB5FE45E7AC1B9AB8D2E94726

WholeHealthMD.com (2005). False unicorn root. In Supplements. Retrieved from http://www.wholehealthmd.com/ME2/dirmod.asp?nm=Reference +Library&type=AWHN_Supplements&mod=Supplements&tier=2&id=7E1C4F4 4E54C42CEB

Wikipedia (2015). Estrogen Dominance. Retrieved from http://en.wikipedia.org/wiki/Estrogen_dominance

Wikipedia (2017). *Resolvin.* Retrieved from https://en.wikipedia.org/Wiki/Resolvin

Wood, R. (2018). Danazol. Retrieved from www.endometriosis.org/treatments/danazol/

Wood, R. (2018). GnRH. Retrieved from www.endometriosis.org/treatments/gnrh/

Wortman, M. & Daggett, A. (2001). Reoperative hysteroscopic surgery in the management of patients who fail endometrial ablation and resection. *Journal of the American Association of Gynecologic Laparoscopists, 8(2),* 272-7. Retrieved from www.ncbi.nlm.nih.gov/pubmed/11342737

Yamanaka, A., Kimura, F., Kishi, Y., Takahashi, K., Suginami, H., Shimizu, Y. & Murakami, T. (2014). Progesterone and synthetic progestin, dienogest, induce apoptosis of human primary cultures of adenomyotic stromal cells. *European Journal of Obstetrics & Gynecology and Reproductive Biology, 179,* 170-4. doi: 10.1016/J.ejogrb.2014.05.031

Yang, Y., Zhang, J., Han, Z., Ma, X., Hao, Y., Xu, C...Zhang, B. (2015). Ultrasound-guided percutaneous microwave ablation for adenomyosis: efficacy of treatment and effect on ovarian function. *Scientific Reports, 5,* Article number: 10034. doi: 10.038/srep10034

Yeager, M. (2016). Adenomyosis: A Significantly Neglected and Misunderstood Uterine Disorder. US: Maria Yeager

Yeager, M. (2012). My Hormones Are Killing Me: Living with Adenomyosis and Estrogen Dominance. US: Maria Yeager

Yeager, M. (2012). The Health Benefits of Omega-3 Fatty Acids in Inflammatory Bowel Disease and Irritable Bowel Syndrome. US: Maria Yeager

Yen, C.F., Basar, M., Kizilay, G., Lee, C.L., Kayisli, U.A. & Arici, A. (2006). Implantation markers are decreased in endometrium of women with adenomyosis during the implantation window. *Fertility and Sterility, 86(3),* S338. doi: 10.1016/j.fertnstert.2006.07.919

Yeung, P., Tu, F., Bajzak, K., Lamvu, G., Guzovsky, O., Agnelli, R.,...Sinervo, K. (2013). A pilot feasibility multicenter study of patients after excision of endometriosis. *Journal of the Society of Laparoendoscopic Surgeons, 17(1),* 88-94. doi: 10.4293/108680812X13517013317833

Yourhormonebalance.com (2018). How Hormones Work. Retrieved from www.yourhormonebalance.com/know-your-hormones/#Progesterone

Zava, D.T., Dolbaum, C.M. & Blen, M. (1998). Estrogen and progestin bioactivity of foods, herbs and spices. *The Proceedings of the Society for*

Experimental Biology and Medicine, 7(3), 369-78. Retrieved from
http://www.cancersupportivecare.com/estrogenherb.html

Zhang, X., Li, K., Bin, X., He, M., He, J., & Zhang, L. (2013). Effective ablation
therapy of adenomyosis with ultrasound-guided high intensity focused
ultrasound. *International Journal of Obstetrics and Gynecology, 124(3),* 207-
211. doi: 10.1016/j.jigo.2013.08.022

Zhang, X., Lu, B., Huang, S., Xu, H., Zhou, C., & Lin, J. (2010). Innervation of
endometrium and myometrium in women with painful adenomyosis and
uterine fibroids. *Fertility and Sterility, 94 (2),* 730-737. doi: 10.1016/
j.fertnstert.2009.03.026

Zhi, X., Honda, K., Ozaki, K., Misugi, T., Sumi, T. & Ishiko, O. (2007). Dandelion
T-1 extract up-regulates reproductive hormone receptor expression in mice.
International Journal of Molecular Medicine, 20(3), 287-92. Retrieved from
http://www.ncbi.nlm.nih.gov/pubmed/17671731

Index

fragarine, 310
free radicals, 92, 134, 200, 306, 385
frequent urination, 127
Frozen pelvis, 136
FSH. *See* follicle-stimulating hormone
funding, 339, 385
fundus, 37
Gabarone, 195
gamma linolenic acid, 282, 298
genistein, 270, 271, 315
ginseng, 300
ginsenoside, 300
GLA. *See* gamma linolenic acid
glucagon, 254
glucose, 75, 77, 78, 91, 255, 322
Glucuronidation, 93
glutathione, 92, 258, 306
glycine, 93
glycogen, 91, 254, 255
glycolipids, 280
glycoproteins, 52, 64
glycyrrhizin, 303
GnRH. *See* gonadotropin-releasing hormone
goldenseal, 197, 301
gonadotropin-releasing hormone, 47, 64, 188, 380, 386, 388
gonadotropins, 64, 368
Gralise, 195
grape seed extract, 92, 189, 301

Graves disease, 84
growth hormone, 85
gynecological surgeon, 137
Haldol, 297
haloperidol, 306
hCG. *See* human chorionic gonadotropin
heavy metals, 215, 307
heparin, 194, 298, 299, 310
hepatachlor, 221
herbicides, 83, 215, 246, 256
herbs, 30, 197, 271, 380, 401
HLA. *See* human leukocyte antigens
hops, 302, 393
Horizant, 195
hormonal balance, 37, 51, 66, 75, 78, 245, 322
hormonal imbalance, 12, 37, 67, 75, 127, 135, 196, 366, 373
hormone replacement therapy, 140, 235, 246, 294, 298, 314, 380
HOX gene, 155
HRT. *See* hormone replacement therapy
human chorionic gonadotropin, 48
human leukocyte antigens, 134
humulone, 302
hydrastine, 301
Hydration, 92
hydrocortisone, 322

junctional zone, 38, 118, 120, 121, 135, 145, 157, 161, 162, 163, 168, 169, 170, 186, 357, 383, 390, 392

junctional zone hyperplasia, 162

JZ. *See* junctional zone

kidneys, 81, 91, 118, 254, 310, 322

Kyleena®, 191

LA. *See* linoleic acid

lactose, 255

laparoscopic excision surgery, 186

laparoscopic uterosacral nerve ablation, 188

laparoscopy, 22, 183, 217, 395

LAPEX. *See* laparoscopic excision surgery

lecithin, 278

leiomyomas. *See* fibroids

lemon balm, 92

leucine, 254

leukotrienes, 99, 104, 306, 366

levodopa, 312

levonorgestrel-releasing intrauterine system, 191, 384

levothyroxine, 309

LH. *See* luteinizing hormone

licorice, 303

lignans, 289, 370

Lindane, 221

Linoleic acid, 100, 282, 358, 370

linseed. *See* flaxseed

lipoic acid, 92, 258

lipoproteins, 280

lipoxins, 99, 101, 105, 366

lithium, 261, 297, 300, 308, 309, 311

liver, 59, 65, 67, 81, 83, 91, 92, 93, 94, 95, 101, 127, 196, 197, 218, 236, 246, 254, 255, 257, 258, 260, 261, 264, 281, 294, 295, 296, 297, 300, 301, 306, 307, 308, 311, 312, 313, 315, 364, 365, 368

LNA. *See* alpha linolenic acid

LNG IUS. *See* levonorgestrelreleasing intrauerine system

Lomotil, 310

Lovastatin, 155, 306

LT. *See* leukotrienes

LUNA, 395, *See* laparoscopic uterosacral nerve ablation

Lupron, 194

lupulone, 302

luteal phase, 48, 51, 63, 153, 316, 370

luteinizing hormone, 37, 47, 52, 316

LX. *See* lipoxins

Lyrica, 195

lysine, 254

rectum, 37, 44, 125, 174
red clover, 311, 393
red raspberry, 197, 310
Reduction, 92
Reglan, 316
relaxant, 310, 316
resveratrol, 262, 390, 391
Retinoic acid, 155
retroflexion, 39, 125
reverse T3, 81
ricinoleic acid, 197
Romidepsin, 155
rosemary, 311, 382
Royal Jelly, 311
s-adenosyl methionine, 312
saliva testing, 237
SAMe. *See* s-adenosyl
   methionine
Sarsaparilla, 312, 313
saturated fat, 278
sciatica, 127
secondary follicle, 47
sedative, 164, 165, 293,
   294, 301, 302, 303, 307,
   364
selenium, 285
senna, 93, 313
serotonin, 199, 254
sex-hormone binding
   globulin, 65
SHBG. *See* sex-hormone
   binding globulin
Silymarin, 306
slippery elm, 93, 314
SLS. *See* Sodium lauryl
   sulfate
Sodium lauryl sulfate, 225

Sorafenib, 154
soy, 233, 290, 314, 315,
   380, 381, 388
speculum, 165, 191
sperm motility, 135
sperm transport, 135, 136,
   389
spontaneous abortions, 146
St. John's Wort, 190, 298,
   312
steroids, 52
stilbene, 262
stimulant, 293, 300
STIP 1, 157
stratus basalis, 37
straus functionalis, 37
stress, 12, 26, 30, 54, 66,
   68, 75, 77, 81, 83, 105,
   139, 157, 179, 201, 245,
   300, 322, 332, 361, 364,
   399
Sulfation, 93
sulfur, 93, 258, 261, 281,
   308, 312
supplements, 30, 80, 91,
   128, 224, 293, 296, 380,
   394, 395, 400
Synarel, 194
synthetic estrogen, 57
T2. *See* diiodothyronine
T3. *See* triiodothyronine
T4. *See* Thyroxine
tacrine, 306
Tagamet, 310
Talwin, 297, 312
tamoxifen, 146, 293, 310,
   314

About the Author

Maria grew up in Cincinnati, Ohio where she became interested in science early in life. She received a bachelor's degree in Microbiology and a Chemistry minor from Eastern Kentucky University. After moving to South Carolina, she became a certified cytogenetic technologist and worked in the field of cytogenetics for twenty years. She went on to receive her master's degree in Holistic Nutrition and a Family Herbalist Certificate from Clayton College of Natural Health. During those years, Ms. Yeager dealt with the pain and suffering of adenomyosis and endometriosis. She dealt with these disorders for seventeen years and only received a correct diagnosis in 2007 when she had a hysterectomy. In 2009, as she stood up from her bed one morning, her right leg gave out. Testing revealed that she had a broken back and herniated disc. This led to three lumbar spinal fusions, two of which failed. Sadly, this led to the end of her cytogenetics career as she was unable to sit for extended periods of time. At that point, she decided to start writing which led to her second career as an author. She is particularly passionate about helping women with adenomyosis and has founded a large online adenomyosis support group called Adenomyosis Fighters. She is determined to do her part in helping other women who unfortunately are forced to deal this horrible uterine disorder. Maria currently resides in Virginia.

Other books by Maria Yeager:

Adenomyosis: A Significantly Neglected and Misunderstood Uterine Disorder (2016)

My Hormones are Killing Me: Living with Adenomyosis and Estrogen Dominance (2015)

The Health Benefits of Omega-3 Fatty Acids in Inflammatory Bowel Disease and Irritable Bowel Syndrome (2012)

Maria's Mixes: A How-to Guide on Making Your Own Herbal Teas (2015)

Life at Nazareth Academy and College, Nazareth, Kentucky (2012)

Blinded by Deception: Life With a Narcissist (2015)

Inspiring Through Experience: A Compilation of Inspiring and Thought-Provoking Christian Blogs (2015)

On Loan From Jesus: The Gift of Little Miss Ally Cat (2012)

62478307R00234

Made in the USA
Middletown, DE
23 August 2019